Develop your Interpersonal and Self-Management Skills

A practical resource for healthcare administrative and clerical staff

Karen Stainsby

Foreword by

Mari Robbins

Radcliffe Publishing
Oxford • New York

Radcliffe Publishing Ltd
18 Marcham Road
Abingdon
Oxon OX14 1AA
United Kingdom

www.radcliffe-oxford.com
Electronic catalogue and worldwide online ordering facility.

British Library Cataloguing in Publication Data

A catalogue record for this book is available from the British Library.

ISBN-10: 1 84619 107 6
ISBN-13: 978 1 84619 107 7

Typeset by Ann Buchan (Typesetters), Middlesex
Printed and bound by Biddles Ltd, King's Lynn, Norfolk, UK

Contents

Dedication

To the memory of my mother, Beatrice, who for many years worked in the frontline of healthcare, and to our good friend, Thomas.

Foreword

A significant development in healthcare over the decades has been the awareness of the pivotal role of medical receptionists, secretaries and other administrative staff. Often, they are the first contact a patient or member of the public will have with healthcare services, whether it be hospital practice, general practice or the private sector. They are the key figures in the field of healthcare, working as part of a team upon whom patients and professionals depend, thus requiring good interpersonal and self-management skills.

This book opens with a comprehensively written section about the importance of effective communication skills, which are essential to good patient care, helping the staff and the public make sense of the many complex systems that may confront them. One must never lose sight of the fact that they may be facing a distressed, anxious, disabled, angry or even abusive person and this book gives helpful advice on how to effectively deal with these situations and to listen first before taking action.

Interpersonal and self-management skills cover a broad spectrum of techniques and approaches, and have a common denominator running throughout – behaviour. Everything you say and do in your dealings with other people inevitably has an effect on the outcome. You know what you are thinking and feeling, whereas the 'other person' only knows what you look like and how you are behaving. This book reminds you about your behaviour in interaction with other people's behaviour. In all of your dealings with other people your approach plays a major part; it determines the impression they form of you and your organisation and the way they react to you.

Karen Stainsby has provided a concise, easy-to-read book, providing essential information that will be of interest and help to new healthcare support staff and those who have been doing the job for some time. It gives helpful tips to understanding the diverse problems and emotions that may have to be dealt with, and a greater awareness of the importance of self-management. It provides a better understanding of the real function of all of us involved in healthcare – personal care.

Mari Robbins
Author of *Medical Receptionists and Secretaries Handbook* (4e)[1]
November 2006

Reference

1 Robbins M. *Medical Receptionists and Secretaries Handbook* (4e). Oxford: Radcliffe Publishing; 2006.

Preface

Closing yet another glossy but worn magazine, I stared up at the clock on the wall and then at the receptionists behind their glass shield. It was ten minutes after my appointment time and my medical ailment remained untended.

My mind wandered back to the time when I too was a GP's receptionist. I remembered the patients who thought that if they stared long and hard enough at us, the GP would hurry up. Then, there was an incident when a patient became incredibly angry and abusive. As she was about to go in for her appointment, the doctor (most inconsiderately in her opinion) chose that moment to rupture his appendix. Having tried to battle on until the end of his surgery, he had failed and was carried out on a stretcher. He was in excruciating pain, she was angry. Happy days!

'Karen Stainsby please' boomed a voice; my turn at last. Ailment inspected, remedy prescribed, I left the surgery happy. I thanked the receptionists and wondered what challenges lay before *them* that day.

I wrote this book to help you in your work role; to provide information and practical suggestions. Although much of the work I have done while working in the healthcare sector has been dealing with the public, the chances are that I have never done *your* particular job. However, I feel privileged to have been told about many, varied experiences while working with and supporting people from different areas within healthcare. So, from what I know, I am betting that a large part of what you do involves communicating with other people: colleagues, patients, relatives, carers and the general public. Given the complexities, vulnerabilities and sometimes 'demanding behaviour' of other people, this may at times be an arduous task. Healthcare jobs take their toll on people, and being able to manage the various demands without being ground down is a great challenge.

The original idea for this book sprang from an informal lunch shared with Maggie Pettifer, the Commissioning Editor for Radcliffe Publishing. We sat at my kitchen table surrounded by the trappings of domestic life. Having never met before, we ate as we swapped stories and experiences from both our professional and personal lives. From time to time we threw in ideas about a book that 'some day' could be written. That 'day' came and you have before you the result of a convivial lunch.

This book is divided into four parts. Part I, 'Communication', introduces the concept of communication: what it is, why it is important, how it goes wrong and how you can help to make it go right. I offer some practical information on the *basic* listening skills that can help us to communicate more effectively. Sometimes it can be difficult to keep a level head and communicate well when under duress and so this section also focuses on handling situations that involve distress, difficult behaviour, abuse, conflict and difference. Part I ends with an exploration of communication using technology, and the pitfalls and complications that can arise.

In Part II, 'Managing yourself', explores some useful skills such as managing time and delegation. Motivating yourself in the workplace can be a real trial, so if you find this an area of difficulty or if you are a slave to procrastination, read this section. Problems, decisions and dilemmas are part of work life, particularly in healthcare where resources may be stretched and the demand high. Part II takes a look at how to handle them.

Part III, 'Working together', begins by looking at team working, what is required to make it go right and what can go wrong. Meetings are a common occurrence at work. The American economist JK Galbraith had rather a cynical view of them: 'Meetings are indispensable when you don't want to achieve anything'. Information in this section guides you through the process of both attending and running an effective meeting. Being able to give (and receive) feedback well is not easy, so I have included some practical advice about this tricky area. Most of us grow up to realise that we can't have everything we want in life. However, we can improve our chances of having *more* of what we want (while maintaining good relationships) by using negotiation skills. Part IV provides much useful and practical information.

Part IV, 'Taking care of yourself', focuses on healthcare's greatest resource – *you*. Despite the medical and technological advances that have occurred, and the work of highly skilled medical, ancillary and support staff, the healthcare sector just wouldn't function without its clerical and administrative staff. This section offers you information about stress and how to recognise and manage it by yourself or with the help of others. Part IV concludes with an exploration of self-understanding: what it is, why it is important to healthcare workers and how to go about finding out more about yourself.

There is also a resource section, which takes you beyond the scope of this book. In it you will find a useful collection of further reading, details of organisations, helplines and websites, etc. This section can be used to further your development or at times when you need an extra bit of help or support.

I have used experiences from my own work and life to illustrate ideas and points. Where case studies do appear, they are based on composite real-life scenarios but do not name or refer to any particular person or organisation.

Some sections will, at different times feel more relevant to the outside world than to work (and vice versa). Nevertheless, we are not divided selves and so what you learn can be applied to either setting. Information that feels less relevant today may take on more significance tomorrow; we never know what's around the corner! At times, this may not feel an easy book to read. It may challenge you, stir feelings, thoughts and memories. While you may be tempted to put it back on the shelf to gather dust, have another go; you might just surprise yourself.

My hope is that this book will help to affirm and build upon what you already know in a way that supports both you and your work.

Karen Stainsby
November 2006

About the author

Karen Stainsby has gained wide experience in healthcare, voluntary, academic and corporate sectors. Her involvement within and on behalf of the healthcare sector spans many years both in frontline and ancillary roles. Over the past decade, Karen has written and delivered numerous personal and professional development courses to nursing, clerical and administrative staff, and others working within the NHS and elsewhere. She has provided support through various change processes within the NHS.

In addition to publishing in the scientific and medical literature, Karen has written articles for *Healthcare Counselling and Psychotherapy Journal* and *Counselling News*, acted as book reviewer for various publishers and editor for *Counselling News*. She has enjoyed several years working as a senior tutor, principal examiner and moderator in the field of counselling and therapy.

Karen now works as a BACP accredited counsellor and qualified supervisor at her private practice in Surrey. When not working, she delights in the simplicity and comfort of family and home life.

Acknowledgements

My thanks go to Maggie Pettifer, Commissioning Editor for Radcliffe Publishing for her initial vision, inspiring discussions and faith.

I am grateful to the many colleagues, patients, clients, trainees and friends, past and present, whose lives have helped shape both me and this book. In particular, I would like to express great appreciation to the numerous healthcare staff who have shared with me both their workplace and personal experiences. I would also like to thank my two colleagues, May Worthington and Helen Hayes, for their assistance.

Thanks especially to Dr David Wicks for his encouragement, editorial comment, technical input and support.

Getting the most from this book

Develop your Interpersonal and Self-Management Skills: a practical resource for health-care administrative and clerical staff has been designed to be used in different ways. One way involves developing an ongoing relationship with its contents in order to aid your professional and personal development. The other way is to call on it during times of difficulty or crisis, when my hope is that it can act as a helpful, reassuring and encouraging companion.

This book is meant to be read in a way that suits you – at the bus stop, sitting in a quiet space or perhaps during a quick tea break. You may be a person who likes to begin at page one and work your way methodically through to the end, or perhaps you prefer to flick back and forth, 'grazing' information. You may choose to apply a lot of thought to one part and merely skim another.

To supplement the text there are boxes entitled:

- *Point to Ponder* – when thinking a little deeper could be useful
- *Experiment* – an invitation to try out new behaviours, plans; etc.
- *A Word of Caution* – when you may need to take a little extra care
- *Tip* – helpful hints.

There are bits 'just for fun' too:

- *It's a Myth* – relevant information that challenges common misconceptions
- *Did You Know?* – a brief, relevant, but little-known, fact
- *Who Said This?* – quotes by famous people (answers at the end of the book).

There are spaces in which to record your thoughts and to make personal notes and comments as you see fit.

How you use this book is up to you. Take from it what you need to move towards a more satisfying life at work and elsewhere.

Part I: Communication

Chapter 1

Good communication

What is 'communication'?

You seldom listen to me, and when you do you don't hear, and when you do hear you hear wrong, and even when you hear right you change it so fast that it's never the same.

Marjorie Kellogg

The ability to communicate, to exchange information, ideas, feelings, hopes, dreams and fears, is perhaps the most influential factor in human development. Grunts and the use of basic body language were how humans began the process of giving each other information. Now, within a matter of seconds, we can talk and write to people on the other side of the world. Messages are sent into outer space with the hope that one day we might communicate with life from other planets and galaxies. People who have undergone massive injuries to their brains or bodies are taught other ways to communicate using, for example, tiny muscle movements. The need and drive to communicate seems paramount to us.

We can't 'not communicate' with others; we do it every day in the way we dress, the use of wedding rings, bindis, tattoos, the car we drive, etc. Good poker players train themselves to keep to an absolute minimum those little tell-tale signs that say 'I have a great hand'.

We are making marvellous advancements in the name of 'communication', and much of what we do is without conscious thought or effort. So why do so many of us find it difficult to communicate effectively? When communication 'goes wrong', so do relationships. 'We don't talk any more' is a very common phrase said to me as a counsellor (most often about partners, but also about friends, relatives, work colleagues and bosses). Perhaps by looking at the mechanism behind communication, we can understand why communication breakdowns occur.

By getting your message across successfully, you accurately convey your thoughts, ideas, etc., to the listener, and they in turn perceive the message in the same way.

Effective communication involves six aspects:

1 the *source*, e.g. speaker, writer
2 the *message*, e.g. words, body language
3 the *communication channel*, e.g. conversation, letter
4 the *receiver*, e.g. listener, reader
5 the *reply*, e.g. spoken, non-verbal reply, written
6 the *context*, e.g. language, culture, occasion, type and history of relationship.

(Adapted from Shannon and Weaver, 1949.[1])

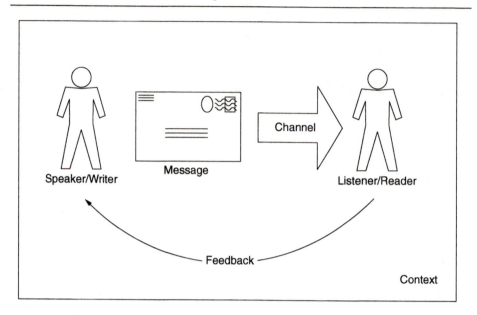

Figure 1.1 The communication process.

A communication breakdown can occur at any point in the communication process. If, for example, I am unaware that the person to whom I have sent a letter is unable to read, my message will not get across. Similarly, if the receiver does not nod their head, smile or even frown when I speak to them, I'm left wondering whether my message has got through at all. Let's look at the sorts of things that can interfere with each part of the process.

1 The source: e.g. the person talks in a quiet voice or chews on a toffee while speaking.
2 The message: e.g. what is communicated and what is left out, what can be read 'between the lines'. Sometimes the message is too lengthy, disorganised, or contains errors, jargon or slang.
3 The communication channel: e.g. bad phone lines, emails sent to the wrong address, talking quietly in a noisy office.
4 The receiver: e.g. ideas and feelings about the message and its source will undoubtedly influence the ability to receive and understand the message.
5 The reply: e.g. verbal acknowledgement, 'I see', nods, smiles or grimaces, email and letter replies, again the receiver's ideas and feelings about the message and its source.
6 The context: e.g. cultural mismatch, failure to appreciate 'newness' of the relationship, wrong thing said for the occasion.

Now we know why and how it breaks down, ways to improve communication include:

• becoming more aware of the communication process in daily life
• noticing the barriers and where and when they happen
• thinking about how to reduce the degree and frequency of these barriers
• using 'listening skills'.

You can learn more about 'listening skills' in the next part of this chapter.

Did You Know?

We 'get the message' from only about 7% of words spoken to us. The rest comes from how we use our voice and body language.[2]

Points to Ponder

- Think of a time when you experienced a 'communication breakdown'. Looking at Figure 1.1, at what part in the communication process did this happen? What might have helped to prevent it from happening?
- Where do you experience most barriers to communication?

Basic listening skills

Nature gave us one tongue and two ears so we could hear twice as much as we speak.

Epictetus

Listening skills are 'advanced interpersonal skills'. They help a person relate more effectively to others, thus building better relationships. These skills can be used anywhere and in almost any situation: with patients, relatives, carers, colleagues, friends, people at home and elsewhere.

But what is the difference between 'listening' and 'hearing'? 'Hearing' means 'picking up sound with the ears', while listening means 'hearing' *plus* 'paying attention'. Listening is a much more complex and active process.

Points to Ponder

- Do you remember a time when someone *really* listened to you? What did they say/do (or not say/do) that helped this? How did you feel?
- Remember a time when you did *not* feel listened to. What did they say/do (or not say/do) that contributed to this? How did you feel?

There are a number of listening skills that you can choose to use in different situations or when you want to achieve certain aims. Sometimes, all you want to have is a short conversation as you make your way to another department, while at other times, a more in-depth discussion may be required, perhaps to explore poor performance or to support a person who is upset. You will already have and use (perhaps unconsciously) some of the necessary skills, while others can be developed. They include:

- reflecting
- paraphrasing
- clarifying
- summarising

- challenging
- immediacy
- self-disclosure
- asking effective questions.

This section will give you information about each skill, why good listeners use it, how it helps and, if misused, how it can hinder the process of listening.

Whatever context or situation, these skills will help you to build rapport and a sense of connection. However, we also know that these skills are more effective when underpinned by three attitudes[3]:

- empathy
- non-judgementalism
- genuineness.

Empathy is the ability to walk in another person's shoes, to see the world how they (not we) see it and to be able to demonstrate this to them. Empathy is different from sympathy, which is more about imagining what it might be like for *us* to be in that situation. Sympathy includes 'feeling sorry' for and 'pitying' the other person. Being empathic requires us to be able to distinguish between what are our feelings and thoughts and what are theirs.

Non-judgmentalism is accepting the person as worthy of being listened to despite what they are telling you. It does not mean that we accept another person's bad behaviour. We all make judgements – it's part of being human – but to enable and facilitate others to talk, we must be prepared to hold our judgements in check.

Genuineness is not 'acting a part' or 'hiding behind' a role (even when you *are* in a role).

Table 1.1 lists some of the specific listening skills.

Three further (and more advanced) listening skills include the following.

Challenging – this does not mean having a fight with someone, but gently raising inconsistencies in what they say or do, e.g. 'Tony, you tell me that you get on well with your colleague Sue, but as you talk about her you clench your fists really tightly.' Challenging should be used only when the relationship is strong enough to take it and balanced with empathy.

Immediacy – again, a skill to be used when the relationship has developed. Immediacy requires the listener to use their own responses to give information to the talker. For example, 'Milly, you tell me that Mike has called you a bully and you say that this is not true. I'm not in your office and so I have not seen how you and Mike interact. However, I did notice just now how loudly you spoke and how close you got to me when telling me about this situation. I felt a little bit bullied myself and I'm wondering whether this is how you come across to Mike?' This skill can be very useful but requires courage.

Self-disclosure – sometimes it can be useful to tell another person about an experience that you have had which may be similar to that being told to you. It can build rapport and may lead the other person to believe that you have an understanding of their concerns. Alternatively, they may worry that their story will upset you and stop talking. They may see your need to talk as greater than theirs. Before giving personal information, ask yourself 'For whose benefit am I saying this?' and 'How will this help Fred to know this fact about me?'

Table 1.1 Listening skills

Skill	What is it?	When to use it	How it helps	Example	Potential dangers
Reflecting	Repeating the same words back	Throughout the listening period	Shows that the listener is really listening	'I am furious at that woman for swearing at me. She has no right to talk to me like that' (talker) 'So you feel furious' (listener)	Overuse can make you sound like a parrot or as if you are not really listening
Paraphrasing	Putting into other words, briefly what the talker has said	Throughout the listening period	Communicates understanding	'I know that I shouldn't get so upset in front of my son but I hate to think that he will have to wait so long for his treatment' (talker) 'That must be a very difficult thing for you; to hide your feelings about your son's illness' (listener)	If overused can interrupt the flow
Clarifying	Seeking more information	When you can't quite see the situation clearly enough	Keeps you on the right track	Can I just check that I've understood you correctly. You've just mentioned a male colleague. Earlier, I thought you said that you worked in an all female office' (listener)	If the story is very confused you may need to use this skill quite frequently. However, you may not need to clarify absolutely everything
Summarising	A brief account that gives the main points of the situation	At the end of a listening period or when you feel stuck or are going around in circles	Helps the talker to feel heard, understood and to move on	'You've told me a number of things today Jackie. Your mother is unwell and your job is very busy at the moment. This means that you can't go and look after her' (listener)	If overused can interrupt the talker's flow

Using questions effectively

Gathering information is another very important part of relating. While it may seem a bit of a contradiction, 'effective listening' involves asking well thought out and skilfully delivered questions.

Depending on what information is required, a listener can ask specific types of questions. Table 1.2 lists some of the more common types.

A Word of Caution

Sometimes when listening it can be tempting to ask a lot of questions (either because the talker or the listener is confused or unsure of what else to say). Too many questions can feel like an interrogation. Try to turn some questions into statements, e.g. 'Don't you like chocolates then?' could become 'I notice that you didn't have any chocolates at break time'.

Sometimes it is not appropriate to speak at all. So how else can we show that we are really listening? We get our body to 'speak' for us. What we do with our legs, arms, head, hands, feet and face will send the message 'Yes, I'm listening carefully to you' or 'No. I'm not interested at all'. The tricky thing about body language is that most of the time, we are unaware of what we do with our body; so we need to be able to notice ourselves more. Remember, body language and what it means will vary between cultures and genders.

Gerard Egan, a psychologist, devised a way for listeners to remember a few simple rules regarding body language. He called it SOLER.[4]

S   Face the person SQUARELY or at a SLIGHT angle.
O   Have an OPEN posture. This communicates that you are open to the talker and to what they have to say. Crossed arms can indicate that you don't want to listen.
L   LEAN slightly towards the talker. This shows interest, but be careful not to invade their personal space and remember cultural and gender differences.
E   Make EYE contact, without staring. Again, be sensitive to cultural and gender differences.
R   Try to look RELAXED (even if you are not). This will help the talker to relax and talk more easily.

Other ways that you can indicate that you are listening include:

- intermittent head nodding.
- saying 'Uh huh', 'I see', etc.
- smiling
- hand gestures
- mirroring the talker's body movement from time to time, e.g. they cross their legs and you cross yours.

Experiment

Begin to tune in and notice the body language that you use in different situations and with different people. What messages might you be sending out? Are they the ones that you want to send out?

Table 1.2 Types of question

Type of question	When to use it	Example	Potential dangers
Closed	When you want single facts or a yes/no type of answer	'Do you like your job?' 'No, I hate it!'	Does not encourage the talker to communicate in any depth
Open	When you want more information	'How do you feel about your job?' 'I hate it. My boss is a bully, the hours are too long and I get paid peanuts!' May open up emotionally charged areas	Encourages the talker to tell you about their situation in more detail which you may not wish to know about or have time to listen to.
Probing	When checking information	'What hours do you work?' '8am to 7pm'	Depending on circumstances, may feel interrogative
Leading	Can aid relationship building and rapport by suggesting understanding	'You don't like working here do you?'	Can be seen as suggesting an answer or advising
Hypothetical	To get a talker to consider new areas and ideas	'What could you do about this?' 'Maybe it's time I looked for another job'	Talker may still be in the stage of telling you about their situation and not yet ready to move on
Rhetorical	When you want to encourage reflection in the other person	'Life's tough sometimes, isn't it?'	Can appear 'clever'

> **Tip**
>
> The more aware you become of your body language and practise using it well while listening, the less mechanical and more natural it will become.

As a counsellor, one question I'm asked often is 'What do you do if a person finds it difficult to talk?' When Marcel Marceau, the famous French mime artist, said 'It's good to shut up sometimes' he was giving good advice to listeners. Many people find silence between two people a difficult thing to handle and feel tempted to 'keep the conversation going'. Also, when time is tight, you may feel like you want to 'move things along'. Talkers stop talking for many reasons, e.g. they don't know what to say, they are thinking hard or they feel very emotional. An empathic look can go a long way, or perhaps a statement such as 'It seems like it's difficult for you to speak at the moment and that's OK' (then shut up yourself).

Another question is 'Doesn't it upset you when someone cries?' Like silence, crying can be difficult to watch if you are not used to it or if it is unexpected. It may be tempting to try to stop a person from crying by pushing a box of tissues into their hands, cuddling them or making kindly meant 'Ssh' noises. Sometimes an attempt to stop someone crying is more about our difficulty with it. Unless there is a good reason why the person *should* stop, crying should be allowed. Again a simple acknowledgement of the other person's distress is enough (either by using a short empathic phrase or a brief nod of the head).

This case study illustrates how people can act with good intentions but fail to listen effectively. 'Mimi' has gone to counselling because she is being bullied by her boss, Gary. During their first session, the counsellor asks Mimi if she has been able to discuss this matter with any of her colleagues. Mimi replies that she has tried and begins to talk about Tina who works in the same office.

> *Tina and I have worked together for a long time and we get on well but I realise that I just can't talk to her about this problem with Gary. Last week things got really bad and I asked Tina if she would come to the canteen for a coffee so that we could talk privately about it. I had been talking for a couple of minutes when I began to cry. Tina jumped to her feet and said that she would go and get us both a biscuit to go with our coffee. When she came back she told me how sorry she felt for me then gave me what she called 'a nice little cuddle'. She does that to everyone who gets upset at work. Then, she told me that she knew just how I felt and began to tell me about the latest problem that she is having with her son! I know that everyone has problems but why, when I just wanted to talk, did it end up with the latest instalment of her domestic drama! I shouldn't talk about her like this; she means well. She started telling me off, saying that I'm too soft and should either stand up more for myself or leave the job. Although I know that she cares a lot about me, I don't really feel like she was listening. I love the job (apart from my boss). I don't really want to leave but I can't seem to sort it out in my head. I'm the type of person who needs to talk about worries out loud so that I can get my ideas a bit clearer and make decisions. My husband, Danny, works things out in his head so he doesn't see why I have to talk to someone. I've got no one else so that's why I've come to counselling.*

Mimi clearly did have people who she could 'talk to' and who did care about her, but things were going wrong in their communication. Mimi wanted to express her thoughts and feelings and for those feelings to be received and acknowledged. She didn't want 'tea and sympathy' or 'a nice little cuddle', but understanding with no judgements attached. There seemed little room for her concerns when Tina's problems became centre-stage. Telling her what she should do and judging her for her inaction made Mimi feel even more inadequate.

Point to Ponder

Can you empathise with how Mimi felt about Tina's efforts to help? If you were Tina, how might you have listened more effectively?

This section contains a lot of information about how and when to use listening skills and it may be difficult to remember it all. Sometimes, looking at what you *shouldn't* do can help to reinforce learning. Imagine that you have been asked to help Penny, a colleague, explore a difficult situation. Having gone into a private office to listen to her, here are 10 ways that you could mess it up (big time).

1 First of all, make sure that *you* are comfortable. If there is only one seat, grab it. Penny can bring in a seat from another office if she wants to sit down. If there is a desk, sit behind it.
2 Do make sure that you sit next to a phone and if it rings, answer it. Even if it's not for you, have a chat; you need a break from Penny and her boring problem!
3 Remember, eye contact is important so make sure that your eyes glaze over after a couple of minutes. This reinforces the message that you haven't got all day and that she'd better hurry up.
4 Use the listening skill of challenging throughout. You will be doing Penny a favour. After all, she needs to realise that people have to be tough to work here!
5 Take the opportunity to strongly disagree and judge Penny wherever possible. Make sure that you tell her what she should do about her problem. You have more common sense than her after all.
6 Do take the opportunity to discuss one of your problems; being listened to is *so* important (and let's face it, you deserve it). Also, this will help Penny to put her less important problem into perspective.
7 If Penny begins to cry, tell her to stop. You should explain to her that 'life is tough' and that it's no use wallowing in problems. If she doesn't stop straight-away, choose one of the following phrases:
   – 'Come here. Let me give you a hug. That'll make it better.'
   – 'Oh, don't cry Penny, you'll set me off.'
   – 'Penny – this is just attention seeking behaviour.'
8 Don't tolerate any silences; they are a waste of your precious time. Make sure that you keep the conversation going, perhaps by talking about yourself (which is always more interesting).
9 In the main, use closed questions. You don't want Penny rambling on forever. Probing questions could prove useful if you want to find out very personal information to tell your friends later.

10 Now it's time to get rid of Penny. Yawn a little, fold your arms across your chest and begin to stare around the room. That usually works but if it doesn't, get up and walk out. Congratulate yourself on a job well done!

Learning to use listening skills is a bit like learning to drive. At first, you have to remember to look in the mirror and be able to change gear while turning the steering wheel. This is a normal phase of learning and the more you practise, the more natural it will become.

Point to Ponder

What listening skills do you already have? Which ones do you want to develop? When and with whom might you go about practising them?

Tip

Desks can act as a barrier to communication. If you must sit at a desk, try to sit 'around the corner' to each other.

A Word of Caution

These skills are very powerful; use them with care and respect. When practising, try them out first in day-to day-conversations before employing them in more delicate situations.

Who Said This?

Which American President was the first to be assassinated and said 'Better to remain silent and be thought a fool than to speak out and remove all doubt':

(a) Abraham Lincoln?
(b) John F Kennedy?
(c) Dwight D Eisenhower?

References

1 Shannon CE, Weaver WA. *Mathematical Model of Communication*. Urbana, IL: University of Illinois Press; 1949.
2 Mehrabian A. *Silent Messages*. Belmont, CA: Wordsworth; 1971.
3 Rogers CR. The necessary and sufficient conditions of therapeutic personality change. *J Consulting Psychol*. 1957; **21**: 95–103.
4 Egan G. *The Skilled Helper*. California: Brooks/Cole Publishing Co.; 1994.

Chapter 2

Communicating with people 'in difficulty'

Understanding strong emotions

Feelings are not supposed to be logical. Dangerous is the man who has rationalised his emotions.

David Borenstein

There is something ... well ... emotive about 'emotions'. Whether they belong to us or to other people, emotions stir and intrigue us. Springing from nowhere and without any conscious effort, we find ourselves in tears while listening to a sentimental song or rousing anthem. Sometimes hard to control, emotions seem like they have a life of their own and a much more primitive quality than our thoughts. Thoughts seem more logical: we can direct them and (usually) make sense of them. Emotion is sometimes seen as the opposite of logic and this can be very frightening. We hear people exclaim 'Look at her! She's taken leave of her senses' as if the person has become someone or 'something' else.

Working in healthcare, supporting ill people and those closely associated with them, you are likely to encounter a wide range and depth of emotions. Some are appropriate to the situation while others may seem quite innappropriate. I remember feeling shocked at the peels of laughter that came from a woman who had just watched her beloved husband die of a heart attack. Having some understanding of the nature of emotions can be helpful to staff involved in frontline care.

The word 'emotion' comes from two Latin words: *ex* (meaning 'out') and *motio* (meaning 'movement'). In other words, we use emotions to express or communicate to others information about our inner state. Our emotions not only help us to communicate with others but also with ourselves. For example, Sally sees a big, snarling dog rushing towards her baby sleeping in his pushchair. Imagining that the dog will bite her baby, she throws herself between the pushchair and the dog. Later, at home, she tells her husband about her 'sheer terror' and he asks whether she was worried that she may have been bitten. 'I didn't think about that. I just did it,' she replied. Sally's emotion of fear communicated to her brain that she needed to do something and in a split-second, super-charged her into action.

Sometimes people use the terms 'emotion' and 'feeling' interchangeably, but emotions are deeply felt feelings, not filtered through the thinking part of our brain. Although we can find many different words to describe our emotions, only five are thought to exist: fear, anger, disgust, sadness and joy. It is interesting that four of these emotions tell us that something *bad* is happening in our life, while only one alerts us to something *good*. Emotions are very primitive and have a universal quality that goes beyond gender, culture, age, race, etc. When someone is angry, most people easily recognise what is being communicated. We learn to do this at a very early age.

Witnessing strong emotions in others can be difficult, and observers respond in many different ways. Some cut off and numb themselves while others over-identify with the other person's emotion and become emotional themselves. At times, it may seem like we are observing something very powerful while feeling powerless to intervene or help.

In the counselling room, some people tell me that they 'never cry'. For them, the fear can be that once started, they will never be able to stop, such is the depth of their sadness, anger and fear. Others tell me that they 'never get angry'. To them, anger has such a destructive force that once unleashed, it will destroy all in its path. Other people use one emotion to cover up what they consider to be a less acceptable one. For example, when Ronnie's 14-year-old son was caught by the police, 'joyriding', Ronnie was angry. Later, when talking to his neighbour about the incident, he began to shake. He realised that much of what he had actually been feeling was *fear* (at the possibility that his son could have been killed). For Ronnie, it was easier to express anger than fear. Such is the power invested in our emotions.

Did You Know?

Our faces have about 90 muscles, 30 of which are concerned with showing emotion.

Our view of our own emotions and those of others will be influenced by our upbringing: what we saw, heard and were told as children. For example, when both a little girl and little boy fall over, the boy is likely to be told 'Get up. Off you go', while the girl is told 'Come here darling. Let Mummy rub it better.'

Points to Ponder

- What are your thoughts about displays of emotion by other people? Do gender, social class, age or culture influence your beliefs?
- Do some emotions feel easier to witness than others?
- Which emotions do you find hard to show? Does it depend upon who is present?

Strange things can happen when we are in the presence of someone who is experiencing a very strong emotion. It can seem as if we 'catch it'. This phenomenon, known as 'projective identification'[1], is different from 'mass hysteria', where one person in a crowd starts to panic and the rest follow. Nor is it the same as 'identifying with' or 'sharing' the emotion. It occurs when a person is so distressed that they find it difficult to experience and express their deep emotion; it is a protective response and easy to understand. It is thought that pre-verbal babies and very young children communicate their needs to their carers using 'projective identification', and we know that an extremely distressed person can become quite child-like. Next time you are with such a person and begin to experience a very strong emotion (for which you have no explanation) it could be projective identification, a 'communication without words'.

Point to Ponder

Have you ever experienced 'projective identification'?

Tip

'When sadness comes, just sit by it and look at it and say "I am the watcher. I am not the sadness", and see the difference,' said Bhagwan Shree Rajneesh, an Indian spiritual leader. We can consider ourselves to be made up of many different parts and do not *have* to identify our whole self with any one emotion.

Who Said This?

Which famous English actress, born with captivating violet-blue eyes during the 1930s, said 'I have a woman's body and a child's emotions':

(a) Judy Garland?
(b) Liza Minnelli?
(c) Elizabeth Taylor?

Helping a distressed person

Anywhere I see suffering, that is where I want to be, doing what I can.

Princess Diana

People involved in healthcare come into daily contact with people who, to varying degrees, are distressed or suffering. How we respond to such a person will depend on our experience of having our emotions handled, messages from our upbringing about having and displaying emotions, and, of course, culture. Being in the presence of a person who is suffering is not easy. This section offers you information on how to recognise signs of acute distress and how to offer help. It is not meant to override or replace medical advice or intervention, departmental policies, protocols or procedures.

Some common signs of distress

People show acute distress in different ways, but some common signs include: crying, screaming, agitation, shaking, inappropriate displays of emotion, disorientation (losing a sense of time and place), depersonalisation (feeling detached from one's own mental processes and body), regression (becoming 'child-like'), unexplained aggression and abusive behaviour. Sometimes there can be no apparent signs at all.

What you can do to help

Remember the first rule of dealing with any emergency situation – ensure your own safety. This may mean different things depending on the situation, e.g. putting some physical distance between you and the distressed person, moving towards a door, asking for the assistance of a colleague, summoning security services and medical assistance. If there are explicit or implicit threats of aggression (to self, you or others) or if you suspect that drugs, alcohol or weapons are involved, do all of the above. If this is not the case, assess whether the person is in a safe place, i.e. not near a staircase or open window (and whether or not they should be moved).

Next:

- assess the situation
- summon assistance, even if a colleague just stands on the sidelines that will support you
- listen to what the person is telling you
- speak in a controlled tone and do not raise your voice
- openly acknowledge their distress
- tell them that you are willing to help
- be aware of your body language and move calmly, slowly and purposefully
- if necessary, drop your body down to their level (but do not crowd them).

A Word of Caution

Know your limits. You might be the first person on the scene but that does not make you wholly responsible.

It can feel very difficult to be with an acutely distressed person. This case study describes a patient, Mrs Smith, and Helen, a receptionist in the x-ray department who attempts to help her.

Last week, Mrs Smith had a mammogram for unexplained breast pain. She had returned to discuss the results with the consultant and, understandably, had felt very concerned. While sitting in the waiting room, she noticed the consultant walk across the room, glance at her and quickly look away. Mrs Smith began to feel even more worried and wondered whether the consultant had some very bad news for her. She started to cry and seeing that she was alone, Helen went to sit beside her. Last year, she had been in a similar situation and tried to reassure Mrs Smith. Putting her arm around Mrs Smith, Helen told her 'Everything will be fine – I'm sure it will'. Later, Helen told a colleague that she knew exactly how Mrs Smith must have been feeling.

> **Points to Ponder**
>
> - Having read the section on basic listening skills, how would you rate Helen's actions and comments?
> - How do you think Mrs Smith might be feeling after Helen's intervention?
> - Might you have done anything differently? If so, what?

Other conditions that can result from extreme distress include panic attacks, disorientation and regression. Each can look quite dramatic so here are some simple ways that you can help.

Panic attacks are linked to the 'fight, flight or freeze' response which primitive humans developed to help them survive daily encounters with wild animals and savage tribes. When panicked, the body prepares itself to deal with the emergency. Blood is diverted from the brain to the parts of the body concerned with fighting, running away or playing dead. As a consequence, a panicking person will find it difficult to think clearly. They may feel like they are losing control, going crazy, having a heart attack or going to faint. Panic attacks last a short time (a few minutes), yet to the panicking person it can seem like an age. Reassurance can be very helpful at this stage. Hyperventilation (overbreathing) can be both a symptom and a cause of a panic attack. Hyperventilating leads to an imbalance in the carbon dioxide to oxygen ratio, reducing the amount of oxygen available to the body. Two strategies can be used to help.

1 Ask the person to sit down. If you have a paper bag handy, ask them to hold it over their mouth and nose (otherwise they can use their cupped hands). They should breathe slowly, in and out of the bag, 10 times then remove the bag and breathe as slowly as possible for 15 seconds. This should be repeated until breathing returns to normal. NB The bag must not be tied around the face nor put over the head and the process must be supervised.
2 7–11 breathing means breathing in for a count of 7 and out for a count of 11, pause then repeat until breathing returns to normal.

A hyperventilating person is likely to require medical assessment in order to assess whether there is any underlying condition that has caused the hyperventilation, e.g. a cardiac problem.

> **Tip**
>
> A panicking person may say 'I can't breathe' or 'I'm choking'. It may help to remind them that a person who is able to *talk* must be able to *breathe*.

Disorientation arises as a way to distance a person from distress. During disorientation, they may temporarily not know where they are, what day it is or who other people are. If it is due to hyperventilation, proceed as above. Alternatively, asking them to look at and name everyday objects around the room can help to 'ground' them. This person is likely to require medical assessment.

Regression occurs when a person returns to a 'child-like' state (another self-protection strategy). You might notice a change in their body language, voice or behaviour. Another common sign is a rocking back and forth or a hugging of the body. Calm but firm reassurance can help; however, as they are unable to take adult responsibility for themselves, they will require medical assessment.

A Word of Caution

It is important to remember that distress may, for some people, be under-pinned by a mental health condition.

After the incident you may need some degree of support (either from yourself or someone else). It may help to talk through with a colleague the thoughts, feelings, imaginings and fears that you experienced and that arise subsequently. You may take the incident in your stride, but occasionally it can be difficult to detach from the experience. You may notice signs that the experience has affected you more than you thought, including reliving the scene, having daydreams and nightmares, and thinking about the person or situation long after they are gone. 'Taking the situation home with you', giving out your home phone number or offering to ring the distressed person at home may indicate that you have not become 'detached'. Talking to your manager, staff support services or occupational health may help. If the situation continues, some short-term counselling may be useful.

Points to Ponder

- How easily can you 'leave behind' emotionally charged situations?
- If you find it difficult, what plans could you put in place that would support you in the future?

Tip

When witnessing another person's distress, remember to breathe slowly, deeply and regularly.

Giving bad news and unwelcome information

> *Ram thou fruitful tidings in mine ears, that long time have been barren.*
>
> Shakespeare[2]

At some time, most people will have been 'the bearer of bad tidings'. Depending on which area of healthcare you work in and your role, you might be responsible for delivering bad news or you might have to do it in a more informal way, when things occasionally go wrong. Perhaps you are the person who has to 'pick up the pieces' after bad news has been given by somebody else. You may just be the first familiar or friendly face someone sees when they have been told something devastating.

Why does giving bad news feel so difficult? When I give bad news, I might:

- have been in the same situation myself
- experience a sense of helplessness
- identify with the other person's upset
- want to give reassurance when there is none
- want to offer hope where no chance exists
- find it hard to choose the right words without sounding clichéd or trite
- worry about the right amount of information to give
- not know what to do with my own distress.

Unwelcome news, no matter how much expected or well delivered, hurts people. This is of course, at odds with the medical principle of 'do no harm'.

The recipient's response can also make the process difficult. While there is no average response, there are some common emotions and behaviour such as:

- a refusal to listen
- denial and disbelief
- anger and hostility
- blame
- an unrealistic optimism.

Point to Ponder

What is your experience of receiving bad news. How were you told? What helped and what hindered?

The *way* that information is given is just as important as *what* is given. Here are some guidelines that may help to ease a potentially difficult process. The degree to which you use them will depend on the nature of the news, the recipient, how expected or unexpected it is and other factors. You will need to use your discretion.

Beforehand:

- think through what you are going to say and how
- think about where you will give the news; do you need more privacy than normal?
- allocate enough time so that the process is not rushed
- prepare the person for what they are about to hear, e.g. 'I'm sorry, I have some information to tell you. You may find it upsetting'
- don't prejudge the recipient's response. What you may consider to be unwelcome news may actually be welcomed.

During:

- 'treat a person as you would like to be treated' is in many ways, a good maxim, but also remember that people react in different ways
- speak clearly and simply with the least amount of technical and medical jargon possible. It can be confusing and seem distancing
- don't give false reassurances, e.g. 'I'm sure you'll have a new date for your operation soon' (unless you can guarantee this)
- try to be aware and in control of your own feelings
- notice your body language. I know that I can fall into the habit of putting my hand over my mouth just before I give someone bad news

- watch the recipient's reactions and body language. This will give you clues as to whether or not they understand and accept (to some degree) what is being said. They may look at you in a blank manner or shake their head in disagreement
- remember that after the initial information the person may not have heard much, so be prepared to repeat and clarify some (or all) of what you have just told them.

Afterwards:

- express regret simply and briefly
- depending on the situation, offer additional sources of information such as writing information down, providing leaflets, other sources of support, etc.
- don't end the meeting abruptly. If you have to leave, give 5 minutes' notice of your departure.

Sometimes, it is not immediately obvious to whom the 'bad news' should be given. The obvious candidate is the person to whom it applies, e.g. the patient. We know that it is not always that clear cut. Is the patient capable of hearing and understanding the news? Do other people need to know as well (or perhaps even before the patient)? Sometimes there are cultural implications. For example, in China, unwelcome news is not usually given to the patient first but to a relative. What do your workplace policies and procedures require and advise?

Point to Ponder

'Who is going to tell her?' he said. 'Not me,' she said. 'Peter can do it. He's the best one at that sort of thing.' Good for Peter, but what happens if Peter isn't at work that day or doesn't want to do it this time? What happens in your department? Do you share the task or is it the responsibility of a designated person?

Occasionally, the 'bad news' involves telling someone that you have made a mistake. While there is an appreciation (by most) that none of us is infallible, no one likes mistakes to be made with their healthcare. A sincere apology often takes the heat out of the situation. A truthful response will help to reinforce an existing good relationship between you, their faith in the organisation and their treatment. Also, it may prevent a complaint.

Point to Ponder

Healthcare jobs can be difficult enough without the added pressure of having to deliver unwelcome news. What strategies could you use to support yourself?

Did You Know?

The messenger who brought bad news was believed by the Ancient Greeks to be responsible for it. Often, the punishment was execution; hence we say 'Don't shoot me, I'm only the messenger!'

References

1 Klein M. Notes on some schizoid mechanisms. *Int J Psychoanal*. 1946; **27**: 99–110.
2 Shakespeare W. *Anthony and Cleopatra*. New Cambridge Shakespeare S. Cambridge: Cambridge University Press; 1990.

Chapter 3

Communicating with people whose behaviour is challenging

Assertiveness

Nobody can make you feel inferior without your consent.

Eleanor Roosevelt

Do you find yourself saying 'Yes' when really you want to say 'No'? Perhaps some people see you a push-over or a soft-touch. Alternately, do they think of you as over-forceful or even a bully?

We develop these character traits at any early age by:

- watching and learning the behaviour of people who were important in our lives, e.g. how our parents handled disputes
- listening to phrases, e.g. 'Don't rock the boat' or 'It's good to think of others first'
- conforming to family rules and norms, e.g. 'Our family always gets what we want – no matter what'.

Our culture influences how we behave too. For example, the British are known for their 'stiff upper lip'. Similarly, when a person bumps into another in the street, it is not uncommon for both to apologise for the incident, even though only one was responsible for the collision. Gender-related messages are important too, e.g. women who speak up for themselves are often termed 'aggressive' (and, as a consequence, labelled 'masculine'). Some societies value the needs of the society over those of the individual, e.g. China, and vice versa, e.g. America (and to a large extent Britain).

Points to Ponder

- As a child, what did you learn about being:
  - overly compliant, patient, long suffering, 'nice'
  - pushy, forceful, getting what you wanted at all costs?
- As a child, how did you learn to get what you wanted? For example, did you discuss the matter, throw a tantrum, sulk, become 'Daddy or Mummy's little treasure', yell loudly or do something else? At times, do you still rely on this tactic?

Assertiveness is the ability to:

- recognise your rights, e.g. the right to offer no reason or explanation for a refusal

- state your opinions, feelings, needs, wants and rights in an honest way
- set limits that feel comfortable to you and make decisions accordingly
- listen and consider the other person's position and recognise their rights and needs
- feel more in control of your life
- not feel the need to resort to manipulation, threats or violence.

Like any skill, assertiveness has to be learnt. This takes time, practice and perseverance. Most of all it takes courage to change the habits of a lifetime and to risk possible disapproval.

Point to Ponder

Look at some of these beliefs about assertive behaviour. Do any of them sound familiar to you? Write in the spaces provided replies that would challenge these beliefs. You can add more beliefs (and challenges) if you have them.

Belief *'If I am assertive...'*	*Challenge*
I will be going against what my parents told me	e.g. I am an adult now with my own life choices
I will hurt people People will see me as hard and cold People will think that I am trying to make myself superior People won't like me anymore	

There are many assertiveness techniques to choose from. Not all will suit you and some will be more appropriate in certain situations than others.

Slowing down

Remember, there is no rule that says that you can't take your time before replying to someone. What sort of a thinker are you? Can you think on your feet or do you need a little time to think before replying? Depending on how much time you need, you could have a cup of coffee or sleep on it. Even disappearing off to the toilet will give you a couple of minutes to think!

Broken record

With the advent of CDs, this may seem an outdated metaphor, but the message is the same. Readers who have played records will know that when the stylus meets a scratch or break in the vinyl, a repetition of lyric or tune can occur. The stylus is said to be 'stuck in a groove'. The broken record technique consists of stating repeatedly what you want or don't want in a calm, direct manner, with the persistence of a broken record and using exactly the same words. You do not justify your decision or do anything else other than repeat yourself. You can use this technique in situations where you are unwilling to do what the other person suggests. Using this technique, you stay focused on what *you* want. This floods the listener's brain with the same message, sending it into a trance-like state. This technique works well but must be used with care, as it can, sometimes seem confrontational. It can be softened by introducing a new lyric, one that shows that you understand how your decision impacts on the other person. For example, 'I know that my decision is going to delay your project Milly, however I am not able to work over lunchtime today'.

Fogging

'Fogging' is useful when you are being unjustly criticised (and most useful when multiple criticisms are being thrown at you). The trick is to find one tiny part of it with which you *can* agree. The critic does not expect to hear that you agree with them and so for a while, is confused, buying you time to think. It may seem like 'giving in', but sometimes you have to 'lose the battle' in order to 'win the war'.

Point to Ponder

How easily are you able to 'lose the battle' in order to 'win the war'?

WHAT

WHAT is another useful strategy when you would like another person to change their behaviour.

- (W) WHAT is happening that you wish to comment on, e.g. 'Tommy, you are chatting quite a lot today.'
- (H) HOW does it make you feel or affect you? e.g. 'I'm not able to concentrate.'
- (A) ASK for change, e.g. 'Please could you lower your voice?'
- (T) How the situation is likely to TURN OUT if there is a change in the other person's behaviour, e.g. 'We'll both be able to finish our work and then we can go and get a coffee together.' Be careful not to use this as an opportunity to threaten, e.g. 'Tommy, if you don't shut up, I'll tell Sally that you are stopping me from doing my work.'

A Word of Caution

Assertiveness is powerful so use just enough to get what you want. You can always call upon more if necessary

---

Saying 'No'

An important aspect of being assertive is the ability to say 'No'. At times, this can be a difficult thing to do, but without it, certain people have a habit of taking advantage, e.g. the patient who insists that they must have an appointment today (despite the lack of a medical emergency). Ask yourself 'Who is running my life?', 'Who is pulling my strings?'

To say 'No' assertively:

1 acknowledge the request
2 say that you are unable to meet the request
3 give a reason (if you want to), but keep it simple (or else you will weaken your case)
4 say 'No' without apologising (unless you have actually done something wrong)
5 suggest an alternative way of them getting what they want (as appropriate).

Tip

While I don't often hear honest apologies, I do hear many people prefacing a refusal with 'Sorry…'; it has become a cultural trait. Notice whether you might do this. Don't apologise unless you genuinely are sorry.

Point to Ponder

Imagine that someone has asked you to do something that you just don't want to do. Write down (or imagine, if that feels easier) a 'no holds barred' type of response where anything can be said. Now, modify your response so that it says 'No' in an assertive manner.

'No holds barred' response:

'..'

Assertive response:

'..'

Sometimes, you might want to get something from someone who doesn't want you to have it. Here are some suggestions that could help.

• First, ask yourself, 'Do I really want this thing?'
• Ask for one thing at a time, using as few sentences as possible. In that way you don't look like you are asking for too much.
• Own your statements by using 'I'. Although you may want to 'pull in the troops', it is much more assertive to say 'I' than 'We'.

Tip

Some people say 'I *need* XYZ' when they actually mean 'I *want* XYZ' or 'I *would like* XYZ'. The motivation behind this seems to be that when we say 'I need...', it carries more weight, more urgency and an implication that if we don't get what we 'need', terrible consequences will ensue. In reality, there are very few things that humans actually 'need', i.e. food, water, shelter and love. Likely to be learnt at an early age, saying 'I need' can sound, well, sort of 'needy'.

When taking an assertive stance, it is important to remember your body language.

- Keep eye contact without staring at the other person.
- Be aware of your posture. Stand upright with your shoulders back and head up.
- Have an open posture, i.e. don't fold your arms across your body.
- Notice any big arm gestures that could make you look aggressive.
- Respect the 'personal space' of the other person.

Some words of warning about being assertive

As you become more assertive, people will notice the change. If previously they have seen you as aggressive, they may be relieved that you are more amenable or they may see you as having lost your 'muscle'. If you have been more of a passive person, they may say 'It's good to see Linda standing up for herself these days' or they may realise that they can't get their own way anymore (and not like it). Most people will like the 'new you', but there will be some who find the change hard to cope with. You may wish to go slowly or to tell people that you have decided to try out some changes in behaviour. Whatever happens, you will like yourself more and the majority of other people will too.

Becoming assertive is a process. It may take some time and you will encounter setbacks, but it is worth doing. As you begin to practise some basic assertiveness skills, you will develop confidence. Don't set yourself up for a fall; in other words, try small tasks to begin with and build on small successes.

Point to Ponder

If you were to act in an assertive manner:

(a) what might you gain, e.g. respect
(b) what might you risk losing, e.g. a passive person may lose being looked after by others?

Experiment

Over the next week, practise saying 'No' to something that you know you would find a bit difficult. Start with something small, e.g. 'I won't have that third cake thank you very much', then build up to a more challenging refusal. Notice how you feel as you 'Say No'.

It's a Myth

We might choose to define ourselves by our gender but that does not mean that our behaviour has to be dictated by the current stereotypes applied to that gender.

Handling angry and abusive behaviour

I know of no more disagreeable sensation than to be left feeling generally angry without anybody in particular to be angry at.

Frank Moor Colby

In 2003, 32% of NHS staff said that they had suffered violence or abuse from patients or relatives. Two years later the figure had fallen to 28%.[1] The reduction is linked to the introduction of the NHS Security Management Service, which took responsibility for tackling the issue of staff abuse in 2003. The survey also highlighted low numbers of staff reporting incidents of violence and abuse.

Acts of extreme violence are rare within the healthcare environment, but anger, verbal threats and abuse are commonplace. Why do patients, relatives and others get so angry?

Anger is an emotion. It is a protestation that something undesirable *has* happened (imagined or real) or *will* happen (no matter how unlikely). People get angry when they feel threatened, frightened or unjustly treated.

Often an angry outburst is underpinned by personal factors. For example:

- ill health
- pain
- stress
- hunger
- tiredness
- hormonal changes (e.g. pregnancy, thyroid disease)
- mental health issues.

Factors external to a person can also lead to angry outbursts.

- Poor communication, e.g. 'You didn't tell me that you were cancelling my appointment until the last minute' or 'Why didn't you tell me that you were going to take £500 out of our joint account?', or gossip, e.g. 'I've just heard that the department is shutting down. You didn't tell me.'
- Insufficient resources, e.g. 'I can't help the queue. There aren't enough staff here today.'

- Bad management, e.g. 'I've told you so many times how Marilyn bullies me and you still haven't spoken to her.'
- Injustice, e.g. 'I was in the queue first. Why was that woman seen before me?'

How you respond to a situation involving anger and conflict is likely to depend on what you learnt about them as you were growing up.

Points to Ponder

- As a child, how has what you saw and heard, influenced your responses to anger and conflict?
- Did you see, for example, conflict avoided at all costs, blazing rows, emotional blackmail, one side always giving in, compromise, negotiation, sulking or violence?
- Did you hear? 'Nice people don't shout' or 'I'm finishing this NOW!' [punch]?

Often, we think of anger as being easily recognisable, but signs of early anger can be hard to spot. Before we know where we are, small disagreements can blow up into conflict situations, but there are clues that you can watch out for. These may help you to prevent the situation from becoming worse.

A person in the early stages of anger may:

- have wider than normal eyes with dilated pupils
- have a slightly reddened face
- show increased physical activity, e.g. pacing
- not listen to others
- interrupt conversations
- invade other people's personal space
- make jokes that may not be overtly offensive but feel 'on the edge'
- make vaguely sexual remarks, gestures and behaviour
- be sarcastic.

As a person becomes more angry, they may:

- become pale
- tense their muscles and shake
- speak through gritted teeth
- raise their voice and shout
- take a fixed position
- use threatening or abusive verbal language, e.g. swearing or offensive language or comments
- use threatening or abusive body language, e.g. invasion of personal space
- make offensive comments about you as a person, your race, gender, age, religion, job role, etc.
- use jokes to threaten violence
- threaten to damage self, others, workplace or employees' property.

To manage a situation involving anger and conflict, you first have to manage yourself. That means being able to tap into how you feel and what you think at any one moment.

Points to Ponder

- What signs of anger (a) frighten and (b) irritate you?
- How might you respond?
- Is your response likely to help or to hinder the situation?

Here are some suggestions for managing a situation involving anger.

- Remember to keep breathing – when we are afraid or angry we hold our breath.
- Talk and act in a calm, firm and confident manner.
- Maintain eye contact (but not in a confrontational way).
- Nod your head so that the other person knows that you are listening to them.
- Acknowledge their feelings.
- Don't judge what they are saying.
- Don't touch them. It may lead to a physical attack on you.
- If the person is shouting, talk slightly more quietly than you normally would. A common response is for the other person to drop their voice in response.
- Show them that you are interested in resolving the situation by (a) telling them that you want to resolve it and (b) asking them questions that will help to achieve this.
- Keep focusing on resolving the problem *together*.
- Try not to retaliate.

Abusive behaviour can be handled in three different ways. You can focus on:

- the behaviour, e.g. 'I am not prepared to listen to this swearing' or 'I will walk away if you continue to use that language'. This leaves the person in no doubt that you mean business, although they may see it as confontational.
- the issue, e.g. 'I'm going to see how I can reduce the wait for you'. This ignores the bad behaviour (which can come as a shock to the badly behaved person as they may be expecting to be told off). The downside is that it may suggest that abusive behaviour is tolerated or even helpful when you want to get your own way
- the behaviour and the issue, e.g. 'Please stop swearing at me. Then I can concentrate on working out how to reduce your wait'.

In general, which option would you feel most comfortable using?

Tips

- Remember that all behaviour is about communication. Ask yourself, 'What is this person trying to communicate?'
- I have seen some people use humour successfully to defuse an angry situation. If humour is your strength all well and good. Be careful that a genuine attempt to help the situation is not interpreted as sarcasm or teasing.
- As long as they are not harming themselves, others or property, it may be advisable to allow the person to express their anger for 20–30 seconds (after which time they will probably burn themselves out). If you interrupt them, they are likely to start again.

> • If you feel like blowing your top and you can't contain yourself any longer, walk away, go to the toilet, anywhere.

Very importantly:

• remember where your limits and responsibilities lie. Call for support when necessary
• be prepared to walk away if necessary. You do not need to stay in an abusive scenario.

If you think that you are about to be attacked, remember the flavour enhancer MSG:

(M)   MOVE away
(S)   SHOUT for help
(G)   GET a colleague to call security.

What to do after a situation has involved extreme anger or abuse

It's not pleasant to be on the receiving end of such treatment. Your 'fight, flight or freeze' reaction will have been activated, which means that your body will be flooded with adrenaline and other chemicals related to the stress response. Take some time to calm yourself by employing 7–11 breathing (breathing in for a count of 7 and out for a count of 11).

Depending on the incident, you may be required to complete an incident form. It is the responsibility of any member of staff involved in an incident with a violent or abusive person to ensure an incident form is completed as soon as possible. This helps to protect you and others in future, e.g. by helping to improve existing systems, procedures, protocols, policies, the work environment and training. Your report may be needed in cases of patient exclusion or prosecution.

> **Tip**
>
> Wherever possible, include witness statements in incident reports.

Filling out this report will also help you to 'emotionally relocate' the incident. Sometimes it is difficult to do that and if you are not finding it easy to leave the incident behind, you may benefit from talking to the staff support department, occupational health department, your own GP or a counsellor.

If a conflict situation involves you and a colleague, ask yourself the following questions.

• Can we sort this out with a discussion?
• Can we agree to disagree (and move on)?
• Would it be useful to involve another colleague?
• Should I involve management at this stage?
• Does the situation require me to consult departmental policies and procedures, e.g. in the case of bullying or discrimination?

If you have reached stalemate and see no way forward, calling someone in who can act as mediator can be useful. Mediators help by establishing ground rules for effective communication. They increase interest in resolving the conflict situation in a 'win/win' rather than 'win/lose' way. Mediators help you to plan for better communication in the future.

Tip

In a conflict situation, your mind is likely to launch your body into a 'fight, flight or freeze' response. When this happens, blood is diverted from your brain and you are likely to think less clearly. You may find it useful to develop and practise some short phrases that you could use in a such situations.

Points to Ponder

- What plans do you and colleagues have in place in order to support and protect each other?
- Are you up to date with policies and procedures regarding the handling of abusive situations and harassment?

Tips

- If a colleague is involved in a conflict situation, support can be offered and the level of conflict potentially reduced by silently standing 'shoulder to shoulder' with your colleague.
- Questions beginning with 'Why' can make people feel like they are being forced to justify themselves. 'Why did you come late for your appointment again?' could be turned into a statement: 'You have come late for your appointment for the third time, Mrs Ali.'

Reference

1 Healthcare Commission. *National Survey of NHS Staff 2005*. Birmingham: Aston University; 2006.

Chapter 4

Communicating when there is a difference

Difference and diversity

> *I'm free of all prejudices. I hate everyone equally.*
>
> WC Fields

Britain has been called a 'multicultural society', but what does that mean? Culture is how we organise ourselves. It is a shared system of beliefs, traditions, values, norms, standards, rules, behaviours, attitudes and symbols. The people who create, share and shape a culture may be linked by history, location, language, social class, race, religion, physical ability, gender, political views – all sorts of things. Our culture need not be fixed in stone; it is influenced by various aspects of life, including social, economic and political factors.

Each family has its own unique culture (which may be very different from that of the family next door even though both have lived in the same village for many years). It can be easy to think of our own family culture as the 'norm'. As a counsellor, I meet many people who grew up in a family culture that was both damaged and damaging, but to the children growing up within that culture it was 'the norm'.

Our sense of who we are arises from the different life experiences that we have, our unique family system and the messages, rules, values and attitudes promoted by it.

Points to Ponder

- Think about your family of origin (or your current family). What words or phrases would you use to describe your family's culture, e.g. competitive, chaotic, safe? Bear in mind that family 'in jokes' and catchphrases can also reveal much about a family culture. Can you recall any?
- Alternatively, think about the office or department in which you work. How would you describe the culture that exists there?

Amidst this diversity, what we share is our almost universal discomfort with difference. As a general rule, there are two ways that we can look at difference. Either we 'see' a similarity between ourselves and other people (even when it doesn't exist) or we become very aware of any difference.

Being in contact with people from different cultures impacts on and challenges our thoughts, behaviours and emotions. We feel challenged because the values, ideas, beliefs and behaviours may be very different from our own, leading to a loss of the familiar, the safe (all of which may not be conscious). When a person leaves their own culture and becomes involved in another very different one (perhaps becoming the minority) they can experience 'culture shock'.

As there is a lot written and spoken about 'difference', it may be useful to clarify the meaning of some of the words that you may read or hear.

- *Diversity* – difference or variety.
- *Cultural diversity* – the existence of different cultures within one group or place.
- *Race* – distinguishing physical aspects passed down through the generations, e.g. skin colour or height.
- *Ethnicity* – a psychological state and, by definition, a more changeable state, e.g. language use, religion.
- *Ethnocentrism* – the belief that your own nation, culture or group is 'central' and is more important, superior, has higher status or is valued more than others.
- *Stereotype* – an idea, attitude or belief held by one group about another as 'fact'. Stereotyped thinking is characterised by simplification, exaggeration and generalisation. Stereotypes are learnt at a time when we think that what we are told by adults is 'the truth' and when it is important, as children, to conform to their views. Stereotypes give us security; if we 'know' who someone 'is' then we feel more safe. They also help us to define who we are (if we are 'not like them'). To justify our stereotypes, we may seek out individuals who confirm it or we may manipulate another person's behaviour to reinforce our stereo-type. This can happen when people hold stereotyped views about us too. For example, a woman whose car breaks down may play 'the lost little girl' stereo-type in order to get her car fixed by a kindly passer by. Alternatively, a man in a supermarket may play 'the little boy' if he is unsure about shopping and what to buy. In the main, stereotypical thinking is more likely to be negative and can form the basis of discrimination, e.g. 'You can't have X because you are Y'. Common stereotypes include those surrounding a person's gender, sexual orientation, ethnicity, race, social class, profession, religious or spiritual belief, mental ability, physical ability, physical appearance, age and status. Those readers who watched the old *Scooby-Doo* cartoons may remember the charac-ters,: Thelma (the intelligent, but plain young woman), Daphne (the attractive, but unintelligent young woman), Fred (the broad-shouldered, male leader) and Shaggy (the hippy anti-hero). All are stereotypes that have been modified in more recent (and more politically correct) episodes of *Scooby-Doo*. These stereotypes were sent up and lampooned when the cartoon became a film. Occasionally, stereotypes can be positive, e.g. the image of different racial groups living well together in the children's television programme *Sesame Street*.

Points to Ponder

- What phrases can you think of that illustrate the stereotypes attached to (a) men and (b)women?
- What stereotypes have people applied to you? How do you feel about that?
- Have you ever found yourself conforming to a stereotypical role that felt uncomfortable?

- *Stigma* – when a person is disqualified from full social acceptance. When we feel prejudiced against a person or group of people we might stigmatise then discriminate against them.
- *Oppression* – can exist in many forms, e.g. name-calling, jokes, physical abuse, exclusion from various areas, etc. We can display prejudice by the everyday language and phrases that we use.

Points to Ponder

- Without judging yourself, can you think of any 'everyday type' phrases that you use which other people could find oppressive or offensive?
- What do you hear that offends you? Is there anything that you can do about that?

- *Prejudice* – an opinion formed from insufficient facts.
- *Discrimination* – to choose a person or group for superior treatment (positive discrimination) or inferior treatment (negative discrimination). It is illegal to discriminate against people at work on the grounds of: disability, sexual orientation, race, age, gender, religious or spiritual beliefs, membership or non-membership of a trade union.
- *Equal opportunity* – to give equal access, e.g. to services, benefits, education, voting rights, health and social care.

Points to Ponder

- Can you remember a time when you felt excluded, barred or 'on the outside'?
- What was that experience like, emotionally and physically?

Coming back to Britain as a 'multicultural society', can culture be measured? Geert Hofstede, a Dutch expert on interactions between cultures, researched the nations of the world and defined different ways of looking at national cultural characteristics. To each nation, he assigned a score which showed whether a nation showed a lot of this characteristic or very little.[1] The characteristics are as follows.

The ability to *take risks and tolerate uncertain outcomes* versus *safety and certainty*. When I inherited some money, my bank invited me to attend a meeting to discuss what I might do with it. Various options were suggested. These ranged from putting the money into a savings account (which involved little risk of me not getting my original sum back and the likelihood of a small amount of interest) to investing in high-risk companies (where I might earn a lot of interest on my money or I might lose the lot). The question was 'How much risk was I willing to take?' The idea of trust and mistrust applies to nations too. In general, nations that may be more new or recently formed and those that have an ethnically diverse population are more likely to take risks and to tolerate the idea of an uncertain outcome. Older countries that have a less diverse population may prefer to stick to what they know and if they don't know may create a superstition or ritual to cope with that uncertainty. People from these nations prefer traditional methods and like to stick to 'the old ways'. The healthcare environment is a rapidly changing one for employees and patients alike and this may not suit everyone. Of course, risk and uncertain outcome have always played a prominent part in medicine and healthcare. Cancellations, rearrangements, new systems, new treatments, younger-looking medical staff can all be sources of stress to a patient from a nation that likes certainty and tradition.

The *power distance* index is a measure of the extent to which less powerful members of a culture accept the distribution of power. A person from a 'high power distance culture' likes those in authority to show their status and will respect them for doing so. This person will feel more comfortable when there is a clear power structure and where uniforms denote rank. Clerical and administrative staff do not usually wear uniform and so may seem to possess no place in the power hierarchy. Conversely, people from a 'low power distance culture' may find a formally dressed consultant, overpowering.

The *individualism versus collectivism* index measures the degree to which a person regards themselves either as an 'I' or part of a 'We'. Individualistic cultures favour personal achievement over group goals (in sporting terms, a golfer compared to a football team). An 'I' person is encouraged to get what will be good for them (with little consideration for the good of the group), to express themselves and not to have to fit in with, be reliant on or dependent on others. A 'We' person will sacrifice what they need for the 'greater good' and be prepared to give and accept help and support from the group. It is not unusual for patients from some collective cultures to involve groups of family members in appointments.

The *masculinity versus femininity* index measures the degree to which a culture favours what are considered to be the more masculine characteristics (e.g. competitiveness, achievement, aggression) over the more feminine characteristics (e.g. nurturing, negotiation). It is the most misunderstood index because it does not equate to gender. For example, a man from a nation whose culture is 'female' is likely to demonstrate more of the feminine characteristics (even though he is male). People from a feminine nation will have bigger respect for the nurturing aspects of the healthcare worker whereas those from a more masculine culture will value efficiency.

When using any model, it is important to remember that it is just that, a model. Hofstede's theories are not set in stone and are based on research done at the end of the 20th century. Although cultures evolve over time, his ideas are still relevant and respected today. There is further information in the Resources section.

Point to Ponder

Think about the ways that Hofstede looked at national cultural character-istics. Have you ever joined or visited a culture where there was a mismatch between your views and attitudes and those of the host culture? How did you manage that situation?

Experiment

Look around your home. Can you find an object that represents your culture. What part of your culture does it represent? How would you describe this part of you to a friend?

A Word of Caution

Britain has also been described as a 'melting pot' but we must be careful not to fall into the trap of thinking that we are 'all the same now'. Communication goes wrong when difference is not respected. Sometimes, there is a fear of saying or doing the wrong thing when communicating with someone who is culturally different from us. This can lead to being overcautious or overcompensating.

Some ways to improve communication across cultures

- Increase your self-awareness around difference – what do 'being different', 'being in the majority' and 'being in the minority' mean to me?
- Develop an openess to new experiences and a willingness to gain knowledge that will enhance inter-cultural relationships.
- Be flexible (within limits) and adaptable.
- Develop an empathic attitude, i.e. the ability to understand what life might be like from the other person's perspective.
- Without denying the difference between you, look for any common ground on which to build the relationship or aid the interaction.

Experiment

This experiment requires the help of a friend. Ask your friend to take turns with you in saying and completing some sentences. These are about the similarities between you, e.g. 'I am the same as you in that I am a woman who has red hair, likes reading historical novels, is a vegetarian' (whatever it is). Try this a few times. Then, repeat the experiment with aspects of yourselves that are different, e.g. 'I am different from you because I am not married, am an only child, etc.'. Notice whether it feels easier to talk about sameness or difference. What felt safe areas and what felt more risky?

Points to Ponder

- What personal and/or professional development might you want to do on the issue of difference? How could you go about addressing this?
- Supposing a colleague was acting in a way that discriminated against a patient. How would you feel? What might you do (or not do)?

Did You Know?

Less than 10% of the languages currently spoken in the world will still be spoken in 100 years time. Two languages die each week.[2]

Working with communication differences

The more elaborate our means of communication, the less we communicate.
Joseph Priestley

So far, we have seen that communication is a complex business, even under the most simple of circumstances. In this section, I want to focus specifically on communicating well with people whose ability to communicate has been affected by a health condition.

Working in the health sector, you will meet many people who have a different way of communicating. As you know, communication is not just about being understood but about having understanding and creating the correct environment in which to understand.

The ability to communicate is influenced by our ability to speak, make known our thoughts, hear the words, see the mouth form the words and to interpret body language. We then have to make sense of information and formulate a reply. Here are some of the most common health conditions (either acquired at birth or in later life) that can affect communication

- *Those affecting the ability to speak*, e.g. dysphasia or aphasia (loss of the ability to produce or understand language), speech disorder (such as stuttering) and 'oesophageal voice production' following laryngectomy.
- *Hearing impairment*: total deafness or hearing impairment, e.g. trauma, mumps and premature birth.
- *Sight impairment*: blindness or visual impairment, e.g. cataracts, glaucoma and albinism.
- *The ability to make sense of incoming information and/or to formulate a reply*, e.g. stroke, dementia, dyslexia, learning ability, expressive language disorder (characterised by limited vocabulary and grammar skills, especially when understanding tense and time words) and autism.

When communicating with a person who has a communication difference remember:

- the power of warmth, compassion, patience and understanding
- a flexible and adaptable approach works best
- communication with others is a fundamental human need, so bear in mind that a person who has difficulty in communicating in a conventional way may have devised another method
- a person's ability to communicate and to understand may not be connected
- often, the person with the impairment will best know the way for you to communicate with them. They can help you
- if you don't understand something, ask for the information to be repeated or for clarification. Not to do this is a denial of the difference between you
- it is easy, when busy, to 'overlook' the patient who has difficulty with communication and make life easier by talking to their carer. Sometimes a carer can act as an interpreter (enabling the patient to retain the power of making choices), but it is important not to ignore the person 'in charge' of their own healthcare

- the patient may be known to your colleagues. Ask them how they have communicated with the patient in the past. What has helped and hindered?
- medical staff will be able to provide you with more information about the medical condition
- while it is important to apply general knowledge and understanding about a particular communication difficulty, it is important to treat each person as an individual and not to assume that all people who have the same condition, will be affected in the same way. Everyone's response, ability to adapt and coping strategies will vary and be at different stages.

Points to Ponder

- Which communication differences do you encounter in your working day?
- How do you adapt your way of communicating to be more effective with that person?
- Is there anything else that you could do?

Tips

- Bear in mind that simplicity works best. Remember KISS (**K**eep **I**t **S**hort and **S**imple).
- An internet site containing a glossary of medical terms, related to communication disorders, appears in the Resource section of this book.

Did You Know?

'Foreign Accent Syndrome' is a rare medical condition that can follow a severe injury to the brain (such as that resulting from a stroke). While the person maintains the ability to speak in their native language, they do so with an accent normally associated with another language.[3] Recently, the accent of a North-Eastern woman was changed following a stroke into what sounded to others like Italian, Slovakian, Jamaican and French Canadian.[4]

References

1 www.geerthofstede.nl
2 Crystal D. *Language Death. Canto*. Cambridge: Cambridge University Press; 2002.
3 Gurd JM, Bessell NJ, Bladon RA, Bamford JM. A case of foreign accent syndrome, with follow-up clinical, neuropsychological and phonetic descriptions. *Neuropsychologia*. 1988; **26**: 237–51.
4 *BBC News*. 4 July 2006.

Chapter 5

Faceless communication

Telephone skills

Middle age: When you're sitting at home on Saturday night and the telephone rings and you hope it isn't for you.

Ogden Nash

It is hard to imagine a world without the phone. While most of us take it for granted, using the phone effectively can be a tricky and complex business. We humans need to make sense of our world and the people in it. We do this on the basis of what we see, feel, touch, taste, hear and smell. Of course, when using the phone, we can only hear. When information is missing, our brain fills in the gaps to make meaning. Here are two examples. First, imagine a picture of a spotty Dalmatian dog represented only by black spots on a white background. Although there is no outline, our brain makes sense of the bits of information that it does have and we correctly see a Dalmatian dog. The brain is a clever machine but does not always interpret the world accurately or consistently. The second example is often used to demonstrate the idea of an 'optical illusion'. You may have seen the drawing of the woman who, when viewed by one person appears as a beautiful young woman wearing a hat but when viewed by another, appears as a hooded witch. We need to be careful about how we interpret information particularly when we are not in possession of the full facts – such as when we are on the phone.

What does your *phone manner* say about you? When leading a busy life, it can be very difficult to retain a good phone manner! When you pick up the receiver, what sort of impression of yourself and your department do you create? How many of us even think about it as our hand grabs the receiver (for the 60th time that day). So many job specifications say 'Must have good phone manner', but what makes a good phone manner?

Point to Ponder

Think back over the last few phone calls that you have received. How would you describe the phone manner of each caller? Jot down some words or phrases that describe what was good and bad.

Good	*Bad*
e.g. polite	e.g. mumbled
....	....
....	....
....	....
....	....

A few other things to consider when using the phone

When the caller can't see you, does your *body language* matter? Try making two business-type calls: the first while lying on the sofa with your feet up and the next while standing up straight. Notice any difference?

How you *pick up* and *put down* the receiver may depend on what sort of day you have had at work and what is going on in the rest of your life. Sometimes, picking up the receiver in a certain way can become a habit and although a caller will not know whether you snatched it up or picked it up in a more controlled manner, you will and what you say next is likely to reveal which it was. Make sure that the cord is not wrapped around itself or you end up straining your neck trying to speak, or worse still, pulling the phone off the desk with a resounding crash and accompanying scream. When hanging up, hold the receiver for a couple of seconds before replacing it in the cradle. No matter how well the call has gone, if it is banged down before the caller puts theirs down it can sound as if you couldn't wait to get off the phone. This may well be true but not necessarily the impression you wish to create.

Putting a caller on hold seems simple enough, but how often do we let the caller know what we are doing, approximately how long they are likely to be on hold and whether they will be listening to silence, music or a phone tone. When I hear silence, I'm not sure whether I have been cut off or should wait a little longer.

Transferring a caller used to be a nightmare for me when I worked in the NHS (quite often I cut people off). In the end, I learnt to say something like 'In case we get cut off, the department/person/extension you want is XYZ'. It can help to reduce the caller's frustration (and the guilt of the person making the transfer). I'm sure you too have had the experience of being passed from department to department or person to person like a rugby ball.

Many busy jobs involve multi-tasking and this is a skill in itself. But how easy it is to fall into the habit of saving time by doing something else while talking on the phone. Being a very sensitive machine, it is amazing how much background noise is transmitted each way (as people who work on help lines will testify).

Here are a few of the things I have heard people from various organisations doing while dealing with my phone enquiry:

- carrying on with their typing
- unwrapping and eating sweets
- interrupting the call to say 'Goodbye' to colleagues
- shuffling papers unnecessarily
- answering a colleague's queries.

Things that I have heard their colleagues doing in the background:

- talking about patients in a derogatory manner
- discussing a patient's medical details (sometimes including their name)
- making personal comments about colleagues.

All of these behaviours left me feeling unimportant, a nuisance for calling or like some voyeur looking into someone else's health records.

> ### It's a Myth
>
> When making an aside, putting your hand over the phone mouthpiece may not prevent the caller from hearing what you say. Not only is it bad practice, but with some systems, your voice can still be transmitted via the earpiece.

> ### Point to Ponder
>
> What phone habits really bug you? Might you have any?

Do you screen calls on behalf of another person? If you are the gatekeeper, I don't envy you. In the imaginations of some callers, you are a fire-breathing dragon who paces up and down outside the cave in which sits the person to whom they wish to speak. What do you say if the person is not available? Here are a selection of phrases I heard this week: 'She's out to lunch' or even better 'She's *still* out at lunch', 'He's not back from lunch *yet*', 'I don't know where he is', 'He *should* be at his desk but he's not', 'I've *no* idea where she is'. I'm sure that in most instances, these gatekeepers didn't mean to give a bad impression of their colleagues (but they did).

Perhaps you work in an environment where you answer colleagues' phones when they are away from their desk. The sentiment behind this is a good one, it means that phones do not go unanswered. But beware the common practice of the colleague who picks up the phone and says one thing while clearly meaning another, e.g. 'Hello, Mary here, picking up Mandy's phone' (*for the 20th time today*). 'She's not here' (*again*). 'Can I help?' (*I don't really want to*). The other common practice is to leave a colleague's phone ringing and ringing until it gets on everyone's nerves when someone picks it up with a 'YES!' (*what do you want!*).

> ### Experiment
>
> Try taping yourself when making calls to five different organisations, e.g. a shop, a friend, the dentist. Play the tape back and notice your phone manner. What do you like about it? What could you change?

Handling difficult calls

Working in the healthcare sector, you are likely to encounter a wide range of caller emotions and tricky situations. While most phones have a 'caller display', work calls usually arrive unannounced (particularly if the majority of the callers are patients and other members of the public). Here are a few of the types of difficult call that you may receive and suggestions on how to handle each.

The hesitant caller

There are many reasons why a caller may be reluctant to begin to speak, e.g. unsure of what to say, frightened that they may say the wrong thing, unfamiliar with using the phone, etc. When this happens, it is best to be patient and use an empathic phrase such as 'It seems like it is difficult to talk at the moment.'

The silent caller

It can be very disconcerting to have someone call you then not speak. Again, there are many reasons for silence, including nervousness, lack of privacy or difficulty with speech. If you feel reasonably confident that the call is not an abusive one, it may help to say 'It's OK. Take your time. If you need to call back, we are here until 5pm tonight.' Sometimes, a silent caller *is* an abusive caller (very common in care-giving scenarios and very unsettling). It is both natural and understandable to say something like 'It's no use not saying anything, you'll have to tell me what you want if you want me to help.' It may be better to take it away from the personal and perhaps say 'The department will shut at 5pm today but will reopen tomorrow at 9am. Goodbye.'

The abusive caller

Abuse over the phone can come in many forms, e.g. the person who swears, throws out personal insults, heavy breathers, those who try to engage you in discussions of a sexual nature (and worse). It is important to know your personal limits as well as your professional ones and to remember that you have the right not to be subjected to abuse. While your first instinct may be to slam the phone down, try not to. The caller is likely to feel pleased that they have had an impact on you. Instead, try to remain calm and remember to keep breathing (as you may hold your breath in shock). Tell the caller in as steady voice as you can muster, 'This behaviour is not acceptable and I am ending the call.' Then put the phone down in your usual manner; this way you remain in control. If possible, talk to a colleague or your manager about what has just happened. While it takes time, it is important to make a record of the incident. First, writing it down will help you to free yourself from some of the emotions, unwelcome thoughts and imaginings that you may be having. If the abuse continues, you may wish to make a case against the caller. Finally, it is important that your organisation is made aware of some of the stressors that you encounter in your day-to-day job.

The long-winded caller

Chances are, when you are at your busiest, the long-winded caller will phone. There are various patterns of long-windedness: some people tell you a lot of irrelevant facts before they can get to the point, while others tell you about their situation over and over again. During normal conversation we gather clues about how acceptable our side of the conversation is from listener's responses but the long-winded caller fails to notice (or ignores) these clues. If you have called someone who you know is long-winded, it is important that you control the call from the start, e.g. 'Mr White, I would like to ask you two questions to help me complete my paperwork regarding XYZ. It will only take five minutes.' Set the limits at the start (and stick to them). Summarise what Mr White has told you and any actions that you have agreed. Ask closed questions to elicit a yes/no response and interrupt if necessary. Much of our upbringing has influenced our abilities to wind up phone calls effectively. Perhaps you were told that it is 'rude to interrupt or not to listen'. As we know, these early messages stay with us and while it may feel easier to make an excuse and end the call, eventually you will run out of excuses to use to the habitual long-winded caller. It may be better to say something like 'I must get on now, Mr White' (which is both friendly and true).

Points to Ponder

- When you were growing up, what messages were you given about listening to other people and interrupting others when they were speaking?
- Are all of these messages still useful to you today? Which ones could you rethink?
- Unpleasant though it may be, imagine yourself taking an abusive call. What types of call would feel difficult for you? What are your personal limits? Write down a few phrases that you could call upon during such a call.

Did You Know?

In the 1870s, Alexander Graham Bell invented a device that could transmit speech electrically. Unfortunately for him, so did fellow inventor Elisha Gray. They raced to the Patent Office and Bell got there first! Hence, we have the phrase 'I'll give you a Bell'.

Who Said This?

Which astronaut said 'The spaceship put in orbit, and the carrier-rocket separated, weightlessness set in. At first the sensation was to some extent unusual, but I soon adapted myself ... I maintained continuous communication with Earth on different channels by telephone and telegraph':

(a) Alan Shephard?
(b) Yuri Gagarin?
(c) Sally Ride?

Email skills

The newest computer can merely compound, at speed, the oldest problem in the relations between human beings, and in the end the communicator will be confronted with the old problem, of what to say and how to say it.

Edward R Murrow

Cheaper and faster than a letter, an email is less intrusive than a phone call and can be sent at any time of the day or night. In the UK, millions of email messages are sent each year and whether they contain vital information or junk mail, all have one aim – to communicate information.

While emails are very convenient, the ease and speed with which most are written and sent can be a problem. Let's look at some of the interpersonal skills involved in writing and sending an email.

How do you begin your emails? Usually, we open a letter with 'Dear' and a phone conversation with 'Hello' or 'Hi', but in email speak there is no agreed convention (nor for closing an email). When replying, it is probably best to use the convention that the sender has used (unless it seems inappropriate to you or to the occasion).

Did You Know?

The first email message was sent in 1965.

In the main body of an email:

- don't use upper case lettering to prove your point. It can feel like SHOUTING (and who wants to be shouted at?)
- don't use too many punctuation marks to push home a point, e.g. 'Who does he think he IS!!??! I am SO ANGRY!!!" (Yes, I think we can see that)
- don't use too many abbreviations (beyond those accepted in common usage such as Dr and Ms). Sentences such as 'Hi M8. Thxs 4 yr msg. CUL8R @ 8 V' may be acceptable between close friends. At best, others may misunderstand what you mean and, at worst, feel unimportant because you have dashed off a reply.

It's a Myth

Emails do not reach the recipient's computer immediately. If you are anxious for a reply, you may need to be patient (and resist the urge to ring up to ask why you 'haven't heard anything back yet'). Email technology has no guaranteed delivery mechanism; the recipient's account may be out of order or switched off by the provider or there may be a network delay. Sometimes, emails just get lost. If a communication is urgent, it may be better not to use email or if you want to know that it has been received and opened, to 'request a receipt'.

When you have written your email:

- read it. Are the grammar and spelling reasonably accurate? Does the tone sound acceptable?
- is there anything that you should add or leave out?
- imagine how the recipient might receive it
- if your email is important or of a sensitive nature, you could ask a colleague to read it before sending.

These measures may sound like overkill, but if your message is important enough to write, it is important enough to get right. A well-written email shows that you respect yourself and the recipient. Consider what impression you are trying to create.

Points to Ponder

- Over the past week or so, have you received any emails that were not well written. What was it about them that bothered you? How could they have been improved?
- What one aspect of your email communication could you change for the better?

Another important point to bear in mind is that email messages do not have the non-verbal expression to add to what is being 'said'. Most of the time we make judgements about a person's emotional state, motives and intentions based on the tone and volume of their voice, body language, etc. When these are absent, it is more difficult to know what is intended and much easier to unintentionally mislead, offend, hurt or annoy someone. Some people have got round this difficulty by using the keys to create 'emoticons' e.g. :-) = happy, :-(= sad. Unless you know how to use emoticons (and you are sure that the recipient knows how to interpret them) they are best left out. Also, the meaning of emoticons varies between cultures.

While on the subject of emotions, it is amazing what people are able to express in an email message – phrases they might never dare to use face to face, over the telephone or in a letter. The speed with which an angry email can be typed and the fervour with which the 'send' button can be hammered both contribute to the email phenomenon of 'flaming'. Flaming can arise from the most innocent of situations too. This is another reason to read emails carefully before sending and on receipt.

If you must communicate your emotion by email, resist the temptation to 'bang out' your message and press the 'send' button with great force. It may be better to go to the toilet, make a coffee or do something else first. When you type it, stick to facts rather than making attacks or personal remarks. You would be wise to ask a colleague to read it before sending.

Email battles easily gather energy and a life all of their own so try not to get into the cycle of receive/send/receive/send. Ask yourself whether you would say to the other person's face what you have just typed? Remember, once you have pressed 'send', it's gone! You may be pleased that you have got your feelings off your chest or you might just hope that your message gets lost! Picking up the phone or visiting your adversary may help to take the heat out of the situation.

It is best not to send an email when its subject:

- requires in-depth negotiation
- is about a disciplinary matter
- concerns a very personal matter.

A Word of Caution

Jokes and cute pictures can brighten up a colleague's day. However, some can take an age to download, cause offence or carry viruses.

A few words about email security

- When talking about a sensitive issue face to face, we use subtle body language which gives clues to indicate just that. For example, we may speak in hushed tones or look left and right as we speak. We may even steer the other person towards the corner of an otherwise empty room. Apart from typing 'Don't tell another living soul' or 'Confidential', this idea is a lot harder to communicate with words. Emoticons can be used but again this requires the recipient to know the convention.
- Unlike a phone call, an email can't be overheard (not in the traditional sense anyway). But do be aware that most organisations have an 'email administrator' with the ability to read all emails irrespective of password protection. It's part of their job.
- Unauthorised people with the right knowledge can intercept and read emails.
- Sometimes emails just go astray.
- If you are in two minds whether or not to send something by email, hand deliver, post it or make a phone call instead.
- Finally, a useful rule of thumb – never send an email that you wouldn't be prepared to have forwarded on to everyone else or pinned up on the departmental notice board.

A Word of Caution

'Phishing' is an attempt to illegally obtain, via email, personal and financial details (usually with the aim of electronically transferring money from you to 'them'). 'Phishers' can appear very credible and may claim to be representatives from your bank or building society. If an email claims to have been sent by your bank, etc., call the bank to verify this. Alternatively, a 'phisher' may say that you have won a prize or offer a large payment in exchange for your financial details.

Did You Know?

No matter how personal your email message is, if you have used your office computer system to write and send it, that document is regarded as the property of your organisation.

Tip

Some people object when their email address appears in a multiple mailing. To avoid this, send the email to yourself and use the 'Bcc' (Blind courtesy copy) facility to send to the recipients. Use 'Bcc' only for this case, as it is easy to press 'Cc' by accident (and send a copy of something to someone who shouldn't see it).

Part II: Managing yourself

Chapter 6

So much to do, so little time

Managing time and delegation

It was a bright, cold day in April and the clocks were striking thirteen.

George Orwell[1]

Time management is a misnomer. How can we manage or be in charge of time – time just exists. The most that we can hope to do is manage ourselves, our attitudes and our behaviours surrounding time. Perhaps a better name for 'time management' would be 'time aware'.

> **Point to Ponder**
>
> When you think of 'time', what phrases come to mind? For example, 'Time is precious', 'Time is money', 'All the time in the world', 'Time is...'

Time management involves three steps.

- Step 1 – What do I want to achieve? Define the goal and identify the tasks required to achieve it.
- Step 2 – How long do I have to do each task? Is the task urgent (to be done as soon as possible) and/or important?
- Step 3 – How do I structure my time in order to complete the task? This is driven by the urgency and importance attached to the task (the time management part).

Table 6.1 shows a simple way to decide.

Table 6.1 Prioritisation of tasks

	Urgent	*Not urgent*
Important	Do now	Do later
Not important	Possibly delegate	Don't do

When focusing on goals, we can use SMARTER to help us.

- **S**pecific – state each goal with a positive statement, e.g. 'My goal is to diet and to lose a stone in weight by this time next year', rather than a negative statement, e.g. 'My goal is not to be so overweight'.

- **Measurable** – if I can't track my success, how do I know in which direction my weight is moving?
- **Agreed** – do I have commitment to this process?
- **Realistic** – can I really lose a stone in a year?
- **Time-oriented** – by a year's time.
- **Everything/body else** – e.g. how does it fit in with family meals and my busy lifestyle.
- **Recorded** – writing down my goal gives me more of a sense of commitment. I stick a note on my fridge door to remind myself.

Tips

- Sometimes it is more relevant and useful to set goals focused on performance rather than outcome. This is especially useful if you don't have much influence over contributory factors.
- Sometimes, a bit of a struggle helps to motivate people. While setting unrealistic goals will probably lead to demotivation and failure, don't set your sights too low either.

What happens when everything needs to be done at once? 'Prioritisation' (or putting 'things in order of importance') will help you. You already use this skill daily. For example, at home, you drop a sharp knife. Down it goes point first. Do you catch it (and risk cutting yourself) or let it fall (only to pierce your new floor-covering)? Both actions have consequences but it all depends where your priorities lie.

Our priorities are based on what we value, e.g. success, personal satisfaction, recognition, as well as our goals, e.g. having a family, getting rich, having a career.

It's a Myth

When he said 'Having lost sight of our goals we redoubled our efforts', was Mark Twain drawing a distinction between busyness and efficiency? Often, 'being busy' and 'getting the job done' are not the same thing.

Here's a simple way to prioritise a collection of tasks. Make three columns, headed *Must*, *Should* and *Could*. Under *Must*, write the tasks that must (at all costs) be done today. Under *Should*, include those that should be done today (but could wait until tomorrow at the latest). In the *Could* column, write tasks that could be done sometime this week (if you can't do them today). Do tasks from the *Must* column first, followed by the *Should* then the *Could*.

Tip

When you have a list of things to do, which do you prefer to do first? Is it the difficult job (to get it out of the way) or the easy one (to get you into the swing of things)? Becoming more aware of your style will help you.

Experiment

Do you know at which part of the day you work best? Are you more likely to accomplish a difficult task in the morning, afternoon or evening (or does it not matter)? As you may know, it's all down to our body clock. Try doing different tasks at different times and see when you 'work best'.

When the goal is large, it can seem difficult to 'see the wood from the trees'. An *action plan* will help you to think and see more clearly what you have to do. It will guide you towards your goal, and help you to monitor progress and to gain a sense of achievement.

A simple action plan consists of seven questions.

Q1   What is my current situation?
A   *I am overweight.*
Q2   How would I like it to be different?
A   *I would like to be one stone lighter.*
Q3   How am I going to achieve this?
A   *By giving up biscuits. I eat a huge amount.*
Q4   What or who could help me to achieve this?
A   *A slimming organisation.*
Q5   What should I do in order to organise this?
A   *Look on the internet for a local group, go along and join.*
Q6   What or who could stand in the way of what I want to achieve?
A   *I have a child and so have biscuits in the house.*
Q7   How could I reduce these factors?
A   *I could ask my partner to put the biscuits up on the top shelf so that I could not reach them.*

Scheduling is the process by which you actively plan your use of time, putting you more in control and so reducing stress levels. It is unlikely that you will be able to remember a more complicated schedule so you'll need something that remembers it for you. Some people prefer electronic organisers (which are great until you ignore the 'battery low' light). Others prefer a paper diary. In the end, *how* you record your schedule is best based on which system you are more likely to use in the long term. There are many types of sophisticated time management systems on the market. However, after an initial flurry of activity, I imagine that many become consigned to a drawer (that one where you keep things that you'll never use again but won't get rid of either).

Tip

When allocating time to tasks and activities, think about football. Each game *should* last 90 minutes but when did you last watch a match that didn't go into 'extra time'? When scheduling, *always* overestimate the time needed to do something (especially if it is for the first time).

I love making a 'Things to do' list. It makes me feel like I'm doing something. But that's just the problem; I 'feel' like I'm achieving huge amounts while getting very little done. Problems arise when I get carried away and my list is made up of largely 'unimportant' tasks. By unimportant, I mean ordinary things that probably would get done anyway. For example, if I wrote a list right now, it would read:

1   buy more shampoo
2   take the washing off the line
3   try to get the ketchup stain off the cushion cover
4   comb the cat's hair
5   comb my hair
6   take the dead flowers out of the vase
7   cut that recipe out of the magazine
8   ring the garage about that petrol leak.

By the end of the day, I am likely to have a great sense of satisfaction. I've ticked off every item (except the last one). Well, I've been too busy – look at my list!

Lists *can* be useful in managing time, but only when the right things are written on the list in the first place.

Sometimes our behaviours 'eat' into our time, chewing it away a little bite at a time.

Point to Ponder

How many of these 'Minute Munchers' visit you regularly and eat your time?

'Minute Munchers'	*Yes*	*No*	*Unsure*
Not being able to say 'No' often enough			
Having a messy environment			
Taking on too much			
Looking at email too frequently			
Insufficient delegation			
Being indecisive			
Not taking risks			
Procrastinating – 'I'll do it later'			
Fire-fighting, i.e. being reactive rather than proactive			
Having unclear goals			
Insufficient prioritisation			
Not having enough information to do the task well			
Not preparing well enough for a task			
Doing something less important			

How many ticks do you have in the 'Yes' column? Perhaps you have identified additional 'Minute Munchers'.

Anyone who has ever worked in an office knows that Sam Ewing, humorist and writer, was right when he said: 'Some of the longest hours of the day follow the question: "Have you got a minute?".' Here are a few ways to avoid interruptions in the office.

- Find out as quickly as possible, why this person has come to see you. That way *you* decide whether you can or should be interrupted any further.
- Be polite but firm, e.g. 'Donald, I'm in the middle of the staffing rota at the moment and will be until 2pm. Could I come to your office then?'
- Visit other people rather than have them hanging around your desk.
- Stand up when someone approaches your desk or say that you need to stretch your legs; that way they are less likely to pull up a chair.

Tip

It is vital that you keep control over ending a conversation. If all else fails and you really can't get away from someone – say you have to go to the toilet. Although it does happen, most people wouldn't follow you in there!

- If you are concerned about being interrupted by phone, use your voicemail, otherwise keep the conversation short and do not be drawn into chit-chat.
- Email technology is another way that someone can interrupt us (if we allow it). When time is tight, pick up, read and respond to email at only set times of the day. Remember just because emails drop into your in tray or 'ping' onto your screen does not mean that you have to deal with them straight away.

Tip

Spam (or junk) email may get through even the strongest filters. If you are getting a lot of unsolicited mail, speak to your IT administrator.

Points to Ponder

- Are you as careful *how* you spend time as perhaps you might be with money?
- What impression do you give about yourself when working to a tight schedule? Do people think that it is OK to disturb you at any time? How 'interruptible' do you appear?

Sometimes, we've just got to give a task or job to someone else to do, i.e. *delegate*. Maybe there is insufficient time in which to do the job ourselves or maybe another person has more of the appropriate skills, aptitude and knowledge required. Delegation is *not* an excuse to dump something that you don't want to do yourself. Nor is it 'passing the buck' to someone else; you retain responsibility at all times. It is a skill to be learnt like any other.

Delegation:

- can bring in new ideas and areas of expertise
- helps you to focus on the bigger picture
- saves you time (in the long run)
- increases colleagues' motivation
- helps the personal and professional development of others
- improves colleague relationships; others feel more trusted and valued.

However, delegation can feel very difficult, for the following reasons.

- A fear of letting go or losing control.
- The need to micro-manage people and situations (as if through a microscope).
- A perceived threat to job security.
- The desire to be seen as indispensable.
- A need to look overworked.
- The perceived threat to authority.
- Reluctance to accept the fact that another person has the skills, knowledge, contacts or perhaps temperament that you don't have.
- Fear that the other person may fail the task.
- Fear that the other person may succeed in the task.
- The 'It's quicker if I do it myself' syndrome.
- The 'no one would do it as well as me' syndrome.
- Difficulty with looking at the bigger picture.

Point to Ponder

Overworked and hassled, it may seem easy to think of giving work away, but how easily can you do it? Do you recognise yourself in the list above?

The *process* of delegation can be divided into seven parts each of which contains important points for consideration.

1. You.
   - What are your motives for delegating the task?
   - Have you the authority to delegate work to other people?
2. The task.
   - Is this task one which could, should or should not be delegated?
   - It is better to delegate 'complete pieces' of work' rather than 'bits and pieces'. People like to see where their piece fits in to the bigger jigsaw and it gives them more of a sense of completion too.
3. The contenders.
   - Who could best do the task? Who has the interest, time, skills, aptitude, knowledge and experience. Who might you wish to develop? Who might have done the task so many times before (or are so skilled) at it, that they would be bored if you asked them one more time.

Tip

It's best to have some idea of the 'person for the job' before setting off to 'prowl' round the office looking for suitable candidates.

---

4. The person to whom you decide to delegate ('Leonie').
   - Is Leonie capable of doing the task (with support)?
   - Is she interested (or would she just be going through the motions)?
   - Is it within her job specification?
   - Do you have to find any resources for Leonie, e.g. people, equipment, training, space?

5 Discussions with Leonie and others.
   – Should you discuss the use of Leonie's time with anyone else?
   – Approach Leonie and explain the job.
   – Why have you chosen her? Tell her how her contribution would fit into the bigger picture. The more she has a sense of 'meaning and purpose', the more chance of success. What will Leonie get out of doing this work?
   – State what you want her to achieve and any constraints, e.g. time.
   – Ask Leonie how she plans (with your support) to tackle this job. Her ideas may be better than yours. Unless your 'way forward' is far better than hers, let her use her ideas. Enable her to voice her opinions, questions, ideas and concerns. If the task is long or complex, it may be necessary to break it down into stages.
   – Agree timescales for monitoring and feedback mechanisms. Leonie needs to know these otherwise she may feel dumped on or abandoned.
   – Check that she has understood everything and that she knows she can come to you if she feels unsure about anything.
   – Inform anyone else who needs to know that Leonie has been delegated the task.
6 Leonie tackles the task.
   – Stand back and let Leonie get on with it! This is the hard bit.
   – Now, you can get on with other things. Yes, you can (this may be why you delegated in the first place.
   – Develop a 'third eye and ear' with which you can follow Leonie's progress, at a distance, as necessary.
   – Appreciate that Leonie may make several attempts at the task before she finishes it.
   – Resist the temptation to look over her shoulder and say 'That's not quite how I would have done it' or 'You could get it done quicker if you did it this way'. Remember, there are many ways to do one task. Review only as and when agreed or if requested by Leonie.
7 Leonie finishes the task.
   – If Leonie has completed the task well enough, congratulate her – it is her success. If she hasn't, you have to look at where *you* went wrong.

Tip

If the task feels so important that you can't resist the urge to micro-manage, the task should not have been delegated or the person you picked is the wrong person.

Twelve golden rules for successful delegation

1 You must have the authority to delegate to others.
2 Closely examine your motive for delegating a task.
3 The task must be one that can *be* delegated.
4 Never delegate a task when your motive is to 'pass the buck' or when you want to prove 'how useless' someone is.
5 You must confer authority on the person to whom you have delegated the task.

6 They must be willing to do the task (otherwise they are unlikely to do it well).

7 Delegate gradually; don't drop people in at the deep end. Even if that's how you learnt, many others have become 'afraid of the water'.

8 All agreements made must be explicit.

9 Watch from afar but keep communication channels open. Unless things are going badly wrong don't interfere – in which case ask yourself 'Why?'

10 Remember, a delegated task does not have to be done as well as you would have done it – just well enough.

11 If all goes well, it is the other person's public success. Privately, you can congratulate yourself on some good delegation.

12 If you have a list of boring or repetitive jobs, don't delegate them repeatedly to one person (usually the one who doesn't complain).

A Word of Caution

Don't delegate if the task involves having a discussion about something very personal, e.g. salaries, promotion, appraisal and review, reprimand, congratulations on a good job done.

Tip

If the task has not been handled as successfully as it could have been, don't fall into the trap of convincing yourself that it would have been better if you had done it yourself.

Who Said This?

Which famous composer, guitarist, singer, performer and satirist, wrote songs for the 1960/70s' band The Mothers of Invention and said 'Without music to decorate it, time is just a bunch of boring production deadlines or dates by which bills must be paid':

(a) Frank Zappa?
(b) Eric Clapton?
(c) David Bowie?

Understanding what motivates you

> *Don't be afraid to take a big step if one is indicated; you can't cross a chasm in two small jumps.*
>
> David Lloyd George

Motivation gets us going, energises and moves us towards goals. It is what gets us out of bed on a cold January morning when the day ahead does not exactly fill us with joy.

Interest and research into motivation really took off following the Second World War, when there was a need to build economies. A few years later, psychologists and managers began to realise that employees were more than just robots; that their ability to work with increased productivity could be influenced.

Various theories for motivation have been proposed.

- We could say that motivation is purely instinctual. Like a newborn baby is motivated to crawl up their mother's body to reach the life-giving milk, so adults have a desire to survive and move forward to satisfy needs.
- Another theory is that humans need a certain amount of excitement in life to feel satisfied and that we will motivate ourselves to find excitement. We all know how difficult it can be to motivate ourselves when the task that lies ahead is boring.
- Do you remember the story of Pavlov's dog (the dog that salivated when a bell rang signalling the imminent arrival of his dinner)? This example of 'conditioned response' demonstrated that dogs (and humans) are motivated by the consequences of previous experiences.
- We learnt, at an early age, to be motivated/demotivated by watching people around us, e.g. parents, peers, those in authority. We watched the consequences of those whose behaviour was either rewarded or punished.

One of the most famous and popular models of human motivation was developed by the American psychologist Abraham Maslow in 1943.[2] Over 60 years later, Maslow's 'Hierarchy of Needs' (Figure 6.1) is widely respected in the workplace and in the field of personal development. His idea was that all humans share fundamental needs (that are arranged in a hierarchy). Once one level of basic needs is satisfied, a person will seek to satisfy more complex needs higher up the hierarchy. The theory rests on one vital rule: higher level needs cannot act as motivating factors unless lower needs are met.

If we apply these human needs to the workplace:

- physiological needs = basic physical needs, e.g. a warm office within a building
- safety needs, e.g. a safe work environment, protection from violence and abuse, job security, safe equipment, existence of rules, policies and protocols
- social needs, e.g. contact and friendship with colleagues, teamwork, cooperation, belongingness, social activities
- ego needs, e.g. recognition, self-esteem, acknowledgement, rewards, respect, status, career development, pay increases
- self-actualisation, e.g. getting the job of your dreams, reaching your potential.

If we have something taken away that satisfies a particular need, e.g. we are moved into an office away from close colleagues, we must meet that need in another way before we can continue clambering up the hierarchy. For most people, the more basic need will always take priority. For example, you may have been concerned that you were allocated a smaller desk than a colleague (an ego need). Later that week, your brother becomes very ill and you can't sleep. Your most basic physiological need to sleep will take priority and the smaller desk pales into insignificance.

Only when our needs are met to a good enough degree can we experience a sense of motivation. But first, we have to recognise and accept those needs, so having a good understanding of ourselves is vital to motivation.

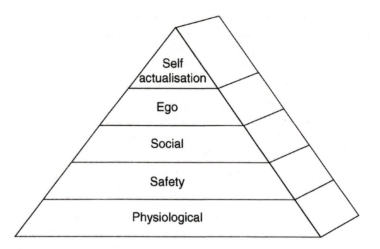

Figure 6.1 Maslow's Hierarchy of Needs.

Point to Ponder

What motivates one person may not be the same as what motivates the person at the next desk and will be determined by factors that include values, principles, ethics, morals, personal philosophy and upbringing. Which of these factors motivate you?

Motivating factor	Yes	No	Unsure
Money			
Interesting work			
Job security			
Common aims and purposes			
Structure (working with rules, policies, protocols)			
The potential to be self-managing			
Teamwork			
Good career prospects			
A sense of belongingness			
Being appreciated			
Being respected			
Being trusted			
Recognition			
Loyalty to colleagues			
Good work/life balance			
Having clear expectations of what your job entails			
Sense of purpose and direction			
Achievable goals			
Freedom to use creativity			
Power			
Authority			
Good working conditions			

- How easily were you able to identify what factors motivate you at work? If you felt unsure about a large proportion of them or certain types of needs, would you benefit from looking more deeply into this?
- How many of your motivators are satisfied by your current job? If there are less than you would like, how could you change things?

Maslow's Hierarchy of Needs is an excellent way to find out what motivates you and what other areas of your life you may want to change in order to feel more satisfaction.

Point to Ponder

Is there another area of your life to which you could usefully apply Maslow's model, e.g. relationships?

Sometimes, finding the motivational energy and getting ourselves going is just not enough. If you are a person who just *keeps* putting things off, then the next section is for you.

Overcoming procrastination

Nothing is so fatiguing as the eternal hanging on of an uncompleted task.
William James

Procrastination is when we put off doing something, e.g. a task or making a decision, until another time. All of us, at some time in our life, use a delaying tactic, but for some people, it can be a real problem.

The word 'procrastination' summons up so many thoughts, emotions and names: 'time waster', 'lazy', 'overcautious'. It carries with it a value judgement.

There are always two sides to the coin. Before we look at how procrastination badly affects some people's lives, let's look at the healthy aspect of leaving things 'until a bit later'. Certainly, if more people 'took a rest', fewer people would be stressed – we are not machines. When we have a list of 'things to do' it can be tempting to race from one completed task to the next without much thought. Often, what we forget (or don't realise) is that the last step of doing anything is to stand back and do nothing except feel the satisfaction of a job done.

Points to Ponder

- What does 'satisfaction' mean to you? How do you experience it; is it a thought, a feeling, a sensation?
- How often are you able to take a step back and feel the satisfaction of having finished a job?

Experiment

Try focusing on an ordinary task, e.g. making a meal. When you have finished, sit back for a couple of minutes and notice if and how you feel any satisfaction? If you don't, how do you stop yourself? What might you tell yourself, e.g. 'It's only a weekday meal, nothing special'? Perhaps you could allow yourself to feel the satisfaction of having completed the task.

Now, let's flip the coin and look at the unhealthy side of procrastination. Postponement of what should be done now harms career prospects, affects and sometimes damage relationships, and robs us of opportunities. 'I wish I had done XYZ. Now it's too late' are some of the saddest words that I hear in my work as a counsellor. Sometimes, there is no second chance.

Point to Ponder

Have you ever procrastinated about something important? What were the consequences?

Before we look at *why* we procrastinate, let's look at *how* we do it. In other words, what crafty mechanism could I use to avoid doing something? I could:

- ignore the task in the hope that it will go away, i.e. the ostrich syndrome
- wait for the right time, e.g. 'It's never the right time to call him'
- wait for the right mood, e.g. 'I've told you, I've got to be in the right mood for that sort of thing'
- hold myself in a constant state of readiness (with the illusion that at any time, I could tackle the task), e.g. 'I've got everything ready to go but I can't make it this week. I'll give you a ring'
- focus on one particular part of the task while ignoring the whole, e.g. 'I'll dust that ornament' (despite the fact that I have to crawl through the debris on the carpet to get to it)
- allow myself to be so overwhelmed by the choices available that I do nothing, e.g. 'I had washing powder on my list but there was so much choice, I came out of the shop without it. I'll get it some other day
- regard a minor setback as ruining the entire task, e.g. 'It's no good. I've eaten a biscuit so my diet is ruined. I'll try again next month'
- do something else instead, e.g. 'I'll just wash my mug up, water that plant and read the paper (because I really don't want to call my sister to discuss our disagreement)'
- have a series of 'little delays', e.g. 'I've got some urgent work to do but I'll just spend five minutes filing these papers, then I'll just make that quick phone call, then … then …'

Point to Ponder

Do you ever use any of these ways to avoid doing something?

Procrastination comes from many sources. It can arise from:

- learnt behaviour – watching the behaviour of other people or getting attention for not getting on with things, e.g. 'I've told you six times, put your school blazer on'
- early messages, e.g. 'Our family always messes it up so it's no use trying'
- lack of organisational skills (including goal setting, time management, prioritisation, delegation and decision making skills)
- lack of self-esteem, confidence and personal power
- a need to hold power over other people by being withholding
- over- and underestimating the difficulty of a task
- difficulty in handling ambiguity and uncertainty
- the need for relevance and meaning in a task or activity
- a sense of being overwhelmed by the choices available
- exaggerated sense of importance, e.g. 'What, *me* tidy out the cupboard!'

Quite commonly, procrastination is rooted in real fear, fear of:

- failure, e.g. 'If I fail, I risk disapproval'
- success, e.g. 'If I succeed, people will think that I am too big for my boots'
- being evaluated or judged, e.g. 'If I don't start then no one can judge me'
- doing something different, e.g. 'But, I've always handed my monthly totals in late'
- commitment
- facing internal anxieties. We can use procrastination to create a drama which then occupies our mind. This directs our attention away from worries such as life, death and relationships.

The bad:bad cycle is a common trap, i.e. 'I haven't done the task so I feel bad. I feel bad so I can't do the task.'

Point to Ponder

Do any of these mechanisms sound familiar to you?

Overcoming heavily entrenched procrastination is not easy. However, a huge step forward is to develop an awareness of it; how, when, where, in what circumstances, with whom and perhaps why you do it. Next you should ask yourself 'Do I really want to overcome it? What are the gains and losses associated with overcoming it?' You may decide that the sorts of things that you procrastinate about are unimportant (and that it wouldn't make much difference if you did sort them out). The pay-off from procrastinating about a particular thing may be too great to lose, e.g. the sense of power and control that I might get from holding up my manager's monthly audit submission. You may conclude that there is a balance between what you would lose and what you would gain. I have included details of a very good book about procrastination (and ways to overcome it) in the Resource section.

Point to Ponder

What sorts of things might you procrastinate about in the workplace? What impact does this have on you, your colleagues, and the service that you provide?

Tip

Remember, the job's not done until you've felt the satisfaction of completion.

References

1 Orwell G. *Nineteen Eighty-four*. Penguin Modern Classics. London: Penguin; 2004.
2 Maslow AH. A theory of human motivation. *Psychol Rev*. 1943; **50**: 370–96.

Chapter 7

Handling problems, choices and dilemmas

Problem solving

'I daresay you haven't had much practice,' said the Queen. 'When I was your age I always did it for half-an-hour a day. Why, sometimes, I've believed as many as six impossible things before breakfast.

Lewis Carroll[1]

The problem with problems is the commonly held expectation that we should be able to get through life with as few as possible (and wouldn't that be nice).

Problem solving is a useful life skill, one with which we are not born. We have to learn how to confront and to handle difficulties without allowing them to overwhelm us. As the Queen of Hearts suggests, this requires practice.

Being in the midst of a problem can feel like being in the middle of a tangled ball of wool or a plate of spaghetti bolognese. This is why strategies have been developed which help us to unravel a situation and see the way forward. Abraham Maslow (he of the Hierarchy of Needs mentioned earlier) said: 'When the only tool you own is a hammer, every problem begins to resemble a nail.' Hence, I offer you a range of problem-solving strategies. Choose which suit you and the problem in hand.

1   Perhaps the oldest and most simple of problem-solving techniques is *trial and error*. This does not rely on finding the best solution to a problem and is useful when you don't have much information or knowledge about the situation. The idea is to try something and see if it solves the problem. If you have taken the right approach to the problem and you succeed – good for you. If you haven't, try something else.

2   *Brainstorming* is a very common way of generating potential solutions and can be done alone or, even more effectively, in a group. The technique involves thinking of as many ways as possible to solve the problem. Its effectiveness can fall down when the 'brainstormers' lose sight of the basic principle, i.e. to generate as many ideas as possible (the emphasis being on *amount* of ideas rather than their *quality*). While brainstorming, it is important to keep the process moving by not thinking too hard, letting your ideas flow and accepting any ideas (no matter how ridiculous). Only when the brainstormer(s) can think of no more options can the list be reviewed and shortened. What remains might just hold the key to solving your problem.

3   Some people find that writing down their problem and 'seeing it in black and white' helps them to find a way through it. Another, perhaps better way for

some, is to draw the problem in the form of a *mind map* (Figure 7.1). Invented by psychologist Tony Buzan,[2], mind maps use words and ideas linked and organised around a central key word. The picture become like a spider. Here are some guidelines to aid the process.

- Use a big piece of paper (bigger than A4). This helps you to move out of 'office mode' and gives your thoughts some room. Write a word or short phrase that represents your problem in the middle. Put a circle or other boundary around it. Draw lines that connect the central theme to your ideas. From these ideas, more ideas will spring. Add them to your mind map.
- Try to work quickly without applying too much thought.
- Don't worry about what it looks like. The aim is not to produce a neat technical drawing.
- Don't judge what you are doing (you can always change it later).
- Use different colours, drawing materials, thicknesses of line, capital letters, numbers, fonts, etc., to make the connections. All will help to stimulate creative thinking.
- If an image or symbol comes to mind, draw it; often, they are more powerful than words.
- If you get stuck down one branch, leave it for a while and move on to another.
- If you can think of other ways that help the process of mind mapping – use them!

4 Because children don't let facts get in the way, their imagination and creativity are limitless, and to a young child, everything *seems* possible. As people grow, many lose the ability to tune in to their imagination, to use it creatively to solve problems. Here are two ways to approach problem solving by using your imagination.

- For some people, ideas are all very good but they are not the answer to the problem. Only when the problem is solved will any value be placed on the 'getting there'. Before that time there will sharp intakes of breath, cries of 'It'll never work' and 'It's no use thinking like that'. Many of us confine our thinking to the familiar and don't consider ideas that may seem a bit wacky or off-key. Developing tunnel vision, we look too much at detail and miss the wider picture. We don't listen to others (even if they may hold the key to our problem), we 'box ourselves in'. *'Thinking outside of the box'* means that we learn to trust ourselves and others more and risk being a little bit unconventional (at least for a while). Developed by Edward de Bono,[3] a Maltese physician, psychologist and mathematian, 'Lateral thinking' is a form of thinking outside of the box; approaching a problem indirectly or by a roundabout route. I have included some further information on this in the Resource section.
- Michelangelo, the sculptor, painter, architect and less well-known poet, had a real gift of imagination. In response to a comment regarding the genius of his latest sculpture, he said simply, 'I saw the angel in the marble and carved until I set him free'. The power of his *imagination* was immense and so is yours. How much are you able to use your imagination? Do you see pictures in your head? Can you lose yourself in a book? If you can use your imagination, then *'visualisation'* may be the problem-solving strategy for you. There are many ways that you can experiment with visualisation.

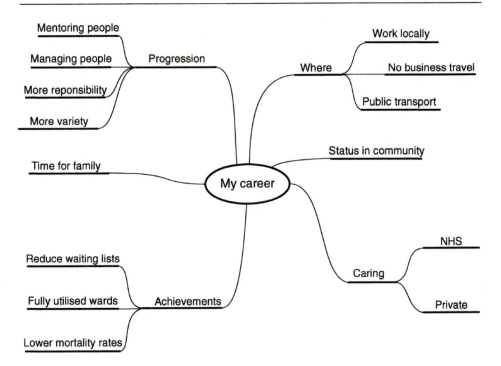

Figure 7.1 Mind map.

I have suggested two scenarios to start you off on your creative journey. Remember, it is your imagination and so you are in control of it. It is best to find a quiet space in which you can shut your eyes, relax and have a few minutes of privacy.

The Jewelled Box

Imagine that you have begun a journey up an ornate, winding staircase. Notice its design, how the banister feels under your hand, how each step feels under your feet. You sit down on the top step and after a moment, notice by your side a beautiful box. It is covered in many different coloured and shaped jewels and locked with a small gold key. You pick up the box, put it on your knee and turn the key. Lifting the lid, you see a folded sheet of paper. Unfolding it, you see written upon it a short phrase. This is the answer to your problem.

The Wise Person

Imagine that you are walking through a comfortable house. Notice the different rooms through which you pass, the sounds, the smells and the noises. Eventually, you reach a room with a big oak door. Opening the door, you see a friendly, wise-looking person who beckons to you. As you draw close, they whisper something in your ear. This is the answer to your problem.

See the Resource section for more information.

Tip

Sometimes, just talking about a problem can help to clarify it. You may not even need to say it to someone else. Have a conversation with yourself out loud; it isn't 'the first sign of madness' and you may just find the solution to your problem.

Point to Ponder

What sort of problems have you faced in your work life? How do you feel you have handled them?

Tip

The 'perfect solution' to a problem rarely exists, usually some compromise is required.

Did You Know?

Lewis Carroll, author of *Alice's Adventures in Wonderland* and *Through the Looking Glass*, was born Charles Lutwidge Dodgson. In addition to being an author, he was also a clergyman, mathematician, logician and photographer.

Decisions and dilemmas

> *One day Alice came to a fork in the road and saw a Cheshire cat in a tree. 'Which road do I take?' she asked. 'Where do you want to go?' was his response. 'I don't know,' Alice answered. 'Then,' said the cat, 'it doesn't matter.'*
>
> Lewis Carroll[1]

> *There is no dilemma compared with that of the deep-sea diver who hears the message from the ship above, 'Come up at once. We are sinking.'*
>
> Robert Cooper

Every day we each make multiple decisions. Some are small and the complications of getting them wrong don't amount to much, while others may have far-reaching consequences. At work, decisions and dilemmas may be fuelled by limited resources and conflicting needs.

Why can decision making feel so stressful?

- When we choose one thing over another, we both gain and lose.
- Even when we decide, there are no guarantees in life.

- We only value the 'right decision'.
- Sometimes, we can feel overwhelmed by the choices available and end up not making a choice.

Choosing is a life skill to be learnt like any other. While some children are asked 'Would you like to choose a sweet from the jar?' others get what they are given. Of course, sometimes out of necessity, children are rushed through the decision-making process, e.g. 'Hurry up, make your mind up. Which cereal do you want? You'll be late for school!' How many anxiety-inducing phrases did you heard as a child, e.g. 'Make sure you choose the right one' and 'No, you've chosen it now. You can't put it back'. Did someone else 'know better' (because they thought that they did or wanted to protect you)? Perhaps you were told that you kept making the wrong choice or were given what felt like impossible choices. Most parents know the trick of 'appearing' to offer choice to a child; either option leading to an outcome desired by the parent (but perhaps not the child). Some children are allowed to make choices but are bailed out when things go wrong. They never learn that there are consequences and that failure happens.

Points to Ponder

- Can you remember making decisions as a child? What messages were you given?
- Turning to you as an adult, what decision-making strategies do you use? Take a look at this selection. Which do you (a) use, (b) use but would prefer not to and (c) wish to develop?

Strategy	I use it	I use it but would prefer not to	I wish to develop it
Take a leap of faith			
Go along with the majority decision			
Be the different one or the dissenter			
Ask someone else to decide for you			
Flip a coin			
Talk to yourself			
Go with your gut feeling			
Really agonise			
Discuss the decision with a good friend			
Decide what you don't want then what remains is the way forward			
Consult your horoscope, psychic, tea leaves			
Ring your friends, think about what they have said and then ring them all again			
Think through the pros and cons			
Refuse to make the decision			
Go for the safe option			
Put the decision off until later			
Put it 'on the back burner'			
Sleep on it			
Put it off all together			

- Have you identified any strategies that you would like to develop? How could you do this?

Point to Ponder

What decisions do you have to take at work? What are the consequences of 'getting it wrong'?

As a counsellor, some people who have a difficult decision to make say, 'Karen, if you were in my position, what would you do?' Perhaps you get asked this too. Sometimes we have to take necessary decisions 'on behalf of' other people. However, it can be easy to over-ride another person's independence in the name of 'saving time' and 'making things easier'.

Point to Ponder

When might you have over-ridden another person's decision or made the decision for them? What were the circumstances that lead you to do this?

Here are some quick ways to make a decision.

- Toss a coin. If your heart sinks at the result, take the other option.
- Write the options on pieces of paper, fold them up and pick one at random. If on reading it, you feel the urge to pick a second piece of paper, this is not the right decision for you.
- Ask yourself: if this decision belonged to a friend, what would you advise?
- Think of a person whose judgement you consider to be good. What would they advise?

A more in-depth way to approach a decision is to ask yourself the following questions.

- *Is* there a decision to be made? (sometimes there isn't).
- Is it *mine* to make?
- Do I have to be make it *now*?
- What are the *options*? Could there be more?
- What credible and reliable *information* do I need to make the decision?
- Should I be talking to anyone else regarding this decision, i.e. those on whom my decision may have an effect?
- What are my *values, needs, wants, goals*?
- What are the *pros* and *cons* attached to each option? Weigh them up.

Tip

If you have a big decision to make remember HALT. Never make a decision when you are **H**ungry, **A**ngry, **L**onely or **T**ired. (David DeNotaris, author, speaker and athlete)

After making a difficult decision, there is usually a sense of relief. For some people this is short-lived and very quickly they begin to feel low. Post-decision sadness is common; whenever we make a decision, we incur the loss of the other option. It can be tempting to 'go back' over the decision and wonder 'Did I take the right road?' Being worried whether you have made the right decision does not make the original decision wrong.

Sometimes, we feel that there is no clear decision between equally undesirable options. We are 'caught on the horns of the dilemma' or 'stuck between a rock and a hard place', both uncomfortable places to be. The following questions may help you when you next wrestle with a dilemma.

- Does either option conflict with the values and principles that I hold?
- Do any guidelines, policies or procedures help me to make the decision?
- What decision would a trusted and respected colleague take?
- Can I justify my decision to myself, a patient, a relative, manager, professional body to which I belong, a complaints board, a court of law? Would they endorse my decision?

What part may *intuition* play in decision making and the resolution of dilemmas? As a small child, my mother often seemed to 'know' things about me in a magical (and sometimes daunting) sort of way. When I asked her how she knew, she would say 'A little bird told me'. I suppose it was easier than saying 'a mother's intuition' (because my next question would have been 'Mummy, what's intuition?'). Today, there is an emphasis on what can be evidenced – the logical, rational, analytical and measurable aspects of life. Intuition is a knowledge not gained by reasoning and intelligence. It is a gut feeling, a hunch, an inkling. Intuition comes from a primitive part of our brain, widely used before we had the ability to think through and analyse situations.

We can call upon intuition when:

- we have to make a decision quickly
- the nature of the problem changes
- information surrounding the problem is conflicting or confusing
- we have never met the problem before so we have nothing on which to base a solution.

Even if we use the conscious, rational part of our brain to formulate the final response, intuition comes from outside of our awareness, from our unconscious. Our intuitive part sees the whole picture rather than bits and pieces. It speaks to us in feelings, sensations, dreams, snatches of melodies in our head and, of course, in the songs of 'a little bird'.

You can best help your intuitive part by giving it as much information as possible and then letting it get on with it. People who use their intuition well, 'put things on the back burner', while others 'sleep on it'. If you have read the section on 'problems' you will remember the idea of using your imagination to help you. You can use the following visualisation when next you have to make a difficult decision. I have called this scenario *The Two Doors*.

The Two Doors

Imagine that you are walking along the oak panelled corridor of an old, comfortable house. On the walls are many different paintings and drawings; take a brief look at them as you pass by. Reaching the end of the corridor, you see two identical doors. Written on both is 'Open me'. You choose one door, open it and pass over the threshold. As you turn to shut the door, you notice another message on the inside of that door. That is the option that you should take.

If the *Jewelled Box* or *Wise Person* scenarios appealed to you, they can also be adapted to aid decision-making.

Point to Ponder

When have you acted upon your intuition? What were the consequences? How could you tune in to your intuitive skills more regularly? Is there scope within your work role to use your intuition?

Things to remember about decision making

- Nobody said that decision making was easy.
- There may be no right or wrong answer.
- Few decisions in life (if wrong) lead to a catastrophic outcome.
- Few decisions are urgent ones, so take your time if necessary.
- You may have made a decision based on the best information available at the time. This is not the same as the *right* decision.
- If it turns out that you have made the wrong decision, take some time to learn from the process.
- Accept that even the best decision makers get it wrong sometimes.

Sometimes we are not the official 'decision maker', but that does not mean that we can't *influence* their decision. Important steps towards doing this include the following.

1 Doing your homework, i.e. gathering information, finding out who is the decision maker.
2 Establishing and building a relationship (or maintaining one that already exists) with that person.
3 Asking the right questions and listening well (to find out information that could support our case).
4 Putting across the benefits of your case (for the decision maker, as well as you).
5 Getting the decision.

The language that we use may weaken or strengthen our case. For example, 'I know that you are not going to like this but maybe, we could…' or 'You couldn't possibly see your way to…' weaken your case, whereas 'Last year, a study on that ward showed that…' or 'This would benefit the x-ray department in two ways' are more likely to strengthen your case.

Acting with confidence (even though you may not feel confident) will help you. Rehearsing your case (perhaps in front of the mirror, a friend or a colleague) will too.

Often, people attempt to give you 'the brush off', but there are ways that you can get round this. For example, if the decision maker says:

- 'We just don't do it that way at St Martin's'

you could say:

- 'What would happen if we did?'

Or if they say:

- 'That won't work'

you could say:

- 'What could we do that could make it work?'

Sometimes, when people want to avoid making the decision, they may say:

- 'Its not my decision to make' – if you had done your homework you would have realised that Mrs Smith did not have the power to make the decision and you should have gone to Mrs Brown.
- 'I really don't know about this Sandy' – what bit don't they know? What information could you give them that would help them to know?
- 'This is not the right time' – find out when the right time would be.

To know *when* to ask for a decision is a great skill; too early and you may look pushy, too late and you could run out of time. Signs that someone is interested in your side of things include: head nodding, leaning forward, genuine smiles, asking for more information and for you to repeat points, checking facts with you, asking you for reassurance, e.g. 'This will be OK, won't it Terry?'.

You don't want all your hard work to have been in vain so make sure that you get a decision.

Point to Ponder

Influencing another person's decision require a good balance of being pushy and holding back. How easily can you achieve this balance when under pressure?

Experiment

Think of one small decision that is not yours to take, but which you know you and the decision maker disagree on. See if you can get them to change their mind.

A Word of Caution

Decision makers have different personalities. You may have to vary the way in which you try to influence different people.

Who Said This?

Which famous American actress and star of *9½ Weeks* said 'I feel there are two people inside me – me and my intuition. If I go against her, she'll screw me every time, and if I follow her, we get along quite nicely'.

(a) Kim Basinger?
(b) Meryl Streep?
(c) Jodie Foster?

It's a Myth

Intuition is not a 'gift' possessed only by 'special people'.

References

1 Carroll L. *Alice's Adventures in Wonderland*. Penguin Popular Classics. London: Penguin; 1994.
2 Buzan T. *The Mind Map Book*. New York: Penguin; 1991.
3 de Bono E. *Lateral Thinking: creativity step by step*. London: Harper and Row; 1973.

Part III: Working together

Chapter 8

Collaborating

Working in a team

Many of us are more capable than some of us ... but none of us is as capable as all of us!

Tom Wilson

Employed within the healthcare sector, you are likely to work within a team, i.e. a group of people organised to work together. Like any other relationship, if a team is to be successful, it must be understood, managed and worked at.

Groups or teams, whether they be a football squad, fire crew, orthopaedic department, prayer group or hate mob, provide a sense of identity, belonging, camaraderie, collaboration, encouragement, respect, challenge, support and a place where we can share information about ourselves. Working in a group satisfies so many human needs. Because we want to continue to have these needs met, we conform to the group's rules, expectations and standards of acceptable behaviour.

The behaviour of individual members and the whole group are influenced by strong, unconscious forces, much of which result from the good and bad memories surrounding that first important group to which we belonged – our family. This is one of the reasons why a group can be a very powerful place to belong.

What makes one group of people work well together and another flounder or be ineffective? For any group to function effectively, attention must be paid to three very different but essential aspects:[1]

1 the *task* or job (often the most emphasised point)
2 the *maintenance* or 'looking after' of the group. A group will not succeed if it does not develop good working relationships
3 the *individual's needs*, e.g. belongingness, recognition, friendship.

Sometimes groups go badly wrong. Let's look at some of the common situations that arise when attention is not paid to the task, maintenance and individual needs of the group.

Scapegoating happens when a group member (usually unjustly) becomes the focus of bad feeling, hostility, criticism and blame. It is a way of shifting responsibility from one or more group members to another member. Often, the person chosen to be scapegoat is someone who is perceived as weaker in some way or is in a minority subgroup.

> ### Did You Know?
>
> The first 'scapegoat' was a goat sent into the wilderness during biblical times. The role of the animal was to make amends for the alledged sins of the Jewish people.

When too many people work on the same task, there can be a tendency for the majority to work less hard (even though the task may require everyone to work hard). So called *social loafing* can result in resentment and scapegoating.

> ### Point to Ponder
>
> Has this ever happened in any groups that you have belonged to?

The departure of a long-established or popular member from a group can raise very powerful feelings within individuals and the group as a whole. Being very primitive in their understanding, the unconscious minds of existing members may regard the new member as an imposter. Worse still, they may see them as having got rid of the person who (as they know at a rational level) retired.

As happens within families, *competition* and *rivalry* between group members are very common. These human traits can be both useful and destructive to the group and the task.

'I feel so guilty now. I just stood there and watched it happen'; the *'bystander effect'* suggests that the motivation to intervene gets less as the group increases in size. This can help to reinforce scapegoating.

A group is happiest when everyone in it shares the same view (even though that view may well be misguided and not held by the majority of members if asked on an anonymous basis). *Groupthink* (a term coined by psychologist Irving Janis) can cause any group to make bad or impulsive decisions, based on little information or selecting only that which confirms the group's view. Disagreement is considered dangerous to the group and the unconscious concern of members is that dissent will lead to exclusion from the group (perhaps by scapegoating or other subtle methods). A good, albeit extreme, example is a collection of football supporters who suddenly (and as if from nowhere), take on a new collective identity and turn violent. In the workplace (and elsewhere) groupthink can reinforce the scapegoating process.

Here are some warning signs that a group is in danger of groupthink

- Individuals keep their opinions to themselves.
- There is an unquestioned belief that the group is right.
- 'Free-thinking police' are self-appointed and often the elders or stronger members of the group. There is pressure on dissenters to think and say 'the right thing'.
- There is an over-rated sense of group togetherness (far in excess of comradeship).

In groups whose primary function is decision making, various strategies have been employed to avoid groupthink. These include anonymous voting and the formal appointment of a 'devil's advocate' (whose role is to argue against group-made decisions). In other types of group, this powerful phenomenon can sometimes be avoided by building up trust and feelings of safety so that members can express individual views.

Did You Know?

Until 1983, a 'devil's advocate' was appointed by the Roman Catholic Church as part of the canonisation process. His role was to suggest that miracles allegedly performed by the potential saint had been produced by more 'human' methods.

All groups go through a *developmental process*, which consists of four definite stages, each with associated behaviours.[2]

1 *Forming* – a time when everyone is 'nice to each other' – members are checking each other out. Anyone who looks like they could be a leader is put in that position (even informally). Questions to oneself include 'Will I be OK here?', 'Who will be my friend?' and 'Who might become my enemy?'. This is the 'vulnerable but cute, young child' stage.
2 *Storming* – the group becomes a battle ground and often there is a fight for opinions to be heard. Issues of power, influence and competition abound. This is the 'stroppy teenager' stage.
3 *Norming* – individuals have progressed through the teenage stage and begin to be interested in working together. There is an emphasis on deciding how to get on with the task and what the unspoken rules of the group are. Mutual support and a sense of getting on with the task emerges. This is the 'young adult learning about responsibility and co-operation' stage.
4 *Performing* – the group is communicating well and getting on with the task in a spirit of collaboration and support. There is trust and members can challenge and support appropriately. This is the 'mature adult' stage.

Like any growing-up process, it does not proceed in one direction for all of the time. If a major event happens in the life of the group, it may revisit an earlier stage before continuing on its developmental path. That event could be almost anything – the loss or gain of a member, a major disagreement or a change in defined roles.

Point to Ponder

Think of a group (in or out of work) to which you belong or have belonged. Do you recognise any of the stages of group development?

In conclusion, for any group of people to work together well, there must be:

- a reason for the group to exist
- a common aim towards which the group strives
- good, honest communication between members
- an appreciation and a willingness to acknowledge differences (not necessarily in an explicit manner)
- enough safety and respect to risk possible conflict

- a good balance between challenge and support
- a collective decision-making process or a formally appointed leader
- an appreciation of how each member's contribution fits into 'the bigger picture'
- flexibility and a willingness to 'help out' when necessary
- a fair division of work
- a sense of loyalty towards the group
- to some degree, an awareness, appreciation and understanding of the strong unconscious forces that act in a group.

It's a Myth

For a group to work well together, it is not necessary that individuals really like each other. They just have to pay enough attention to the group's task, maintenance and individual needs.

Making meetings meaningful

> *Meetings are a great trap. Soon you find yourself trying to get agreement and then the people who disagree come to think they have a right to be persuaded... However, they are indispensable when you don't want to do anything.*
>
> JK Galbraith

Informal get-togethers and chats over a coffee can be very effective, but when issues are more complex, time is tight and decisions are required, a more formalised type of 'coming together' may be necessary.

Does your heart sink when you open your email and notice is given of 'yet another meeting'? Sometimes it feels like you can't get on with your work because you have to go to yet another meeting. I remember frequently being unable to finish work decided upon at one meeting because I had to go to the next one to report on progress.

Meetings, if set up correctly, run efficiently and with the right people, can be very productive. More frequently than not, people 'called' to meetings see them as a waste of time, resources and money. Sometimes, a badly run meeting can create more problems than it solves, leading to a fall in morale and motivation. At the end of a meeting when people say 'Let's get back to work now', you know that the process has not been valued.

Point to Ponder

What is your experience of work-based meetings?

We have meetings to:

- give, receive or exchange information
- discuss issues
- generate ideas
- plan

- get feedback
- find an answer to a problem
- delegate tasks
- sort out or avoid a crisis
- report on performance
- motivate
- reprimand
- set targets
- make simple or more complex decisions
- discuss policy and procedure
- help people to feel more involved
- air differences and heal rifts.

A meeting is a collection of people who come together for a common task. Each person has a role and it is important to know what your role is and what each role does. The main roles are as follows.

- A *scribe* – records the meeting: decisions, ideas, suggestions, comments and tasks to be done after the meeting (actions). It is usual for the scribe to be asked to make a record of the meeting (the 'minutes'). They may be brought in specifically for this task in which case, it is not usual for them to speak (unless something said is unclear or not heard properly).
- An *observer* – watches and pays attention to what is said but probably more importantly, what happens. Their role is a silent one (unless invited to speak by the chairperson). Observers are invited to meetings, for example when there are problems with the way that the group functions or for audit purposes.
- An *expert* – contributes specialist knowledge that the meeting needs to be effective. They may be asked to stay for all or some of the meeting and will not usually be asked to comment on issues outside their specialist area.
- A *participant* – is the 'foot soldier' of the meeting.
- A *chairperson* – is the 'conductor' (more about this important role later).

Some important questions to consider when planning a meeting

Why are we having this meeting?

It is essential to have a clear idea of why you want to have the meeting and what you want to achieve by the end of it. At the end of the meeting, if you hear people say 'Well, it has been really nice chatting with everyone', you will have helped to improve staff relationships (which is great if that was your aim) but very little else. Many people amble along to meetings, not really knowing why they are going but afraid they may miss something if they don't go. A clear aim helps people to feel more motivated to attend.

Who should be invited?

Usually, it is the chairperson who decides (but not always). Knowing who to invite (and who not to invite) can be tricky. Sometimes, not all people invited need to be in the room for the whole meeting; if people think that most of the meeting has been irrelevant to them, they are less likely to attend next time.

The smallest number of participants able to achieve the aim is the right number.

Inviting people from outside of the department, organisation, group, etc., can be useful, as often those not so closely involved can bring a fresh view to a difficult issue. This may not be a good idea if the matter to be discussed is of a sensitive or personal nature. It may be quite appropriate to have members of senior management at the meeting, although at times their presence can feel intimidating. Only invite people who hold decision-making power, can provide specialist information, skills, data or relevant views.

When and where should the meeting be held?

In the interests of both the success of the meeting and human relations, try to find out when all or most of the people can come. Remember that people with childcare and other family and domestic responsibilities may find it difficult to stay to a meeting that lasts into the early evening. Take into account days when staff may not be at work, for example significant religious days. If you take the time to find out these things, people are much more likely to attend willingly and to contribute effectively.

Sometimes, when deciding to have a meeting, attention is focused on the task at the expense of the environment. Where you have the meeting and the facilities that you provide are important. Taking care with this will show respect for the participants and the process. While you will have to work within your means, there are steps that you can take that will help people work better together once the meeting starts. Here are some things I've had to endure which, I am sure, will have affected my contribution.

- Being in an informal setting to discuss a sensitive matter. My concern was that the material may be overheard.
- Sitting in a very formal setting, again to discuss a sensitive matter, but with a desk between us that created a barrier to communication.
- Meeting in an airless, hot, stuffy room with no natural light.
- Badly laid out seating which meant lots of 'neck craning' to read a flip chart.

I'm sure you will be able to add to my list.

How long should the meeting last?

The 'law of diminishing returns' applies to meetings; as the meeting goes on (and on) people concentrate less effectively. I wonder what your experience of meetings has been? At what stage do you typically think 'I've had enough'? When this stage comes, participants 'leave the meeting', in mind if not in body. Taking short breaks, e.g. five minutes every 40 minutes will help participants to remain focused.

Do we always need an agenda?

This depends on how formal the meeting is. The agenda acts as the map to where you want to end up. It helps people to take the meeting seriously. An agenda should contain the following information:

- who called the meeting

- the purpose of the meeting
- what needs to be achieved by the end of the meeting
- who is invited (including outside speakers, guests and experts)
- who is 'chairing' the meeting
- date, time (start and finish) and venue
- apologies for absence
- matters arising from the last meeting (if any)
- approval of minutes of the last meeting (if any)
- matters for discussion at this meeting
- any other business.

The agenda should give information regarding any preparation that needs to be done for the meeting, e.g. spreadsheets, reports. Any papers that should be read before attending the meeting can be attached to the agenda. Agenda items should be ordered in such a way that helps the flow of the meeting. To avoid tiring people, the more 'heavy' items can be mixed in with 'lighter' ones.

Relevant papers or information can be attached to the agenda. It is common (but not good) practice to give supporting information five minutes before the meeting starts (sometimes *at* the meeting). Unless it really is exciting 'hot off the press' news, give it well beforehand.

Even if the meeting is a very informal one, it is a good idea to have a brief agenda in your head.

Tip

While you could take the view that people should (a) not lose their agenda and (b) remember to bring it with them, it is wise to take extra copies to the meeting. If you don't, people will spend their time looking over each others' shoulders.

Do we need to take notes and produce minutes?

Note-taking is about communication. Notes should be written up and a copy given to all participants, plus those who gave apologies for absence. The notes should be brief (if you want people to read them). Names should be spelt correctly and accurate titles and roles given. Good minutes help people to meet actions and stick to agreements.

What is a 'pre-meeting meeting'?

Some people like to have a 'meeting before the meeting'. These can be useful if held between key people who want to thrash out some basic ideas or do some groundwork that would only prolong the meeting unnecessarily. The flip side is that pre-meeting meetings can be regarded (by those not invited) as an arena where everything is 'all sewn up' just to be rubber stamped at the 'real meeting'.

What to think about after the meeting finishes

The meeting may have 'closed', participants left the room, returned to their desks or gone home. But there is still work to be done.

- A record of the meeting (the minutes) should be made, including decisions taken, tasks allocated, date, time, location of next meeting. These are circulated to all participants, those who gave apologies for absence and anyone else who needs to know.
- It is important to think back over the meeting and to ask yourself 'Was the meeting useful?'
  - Did we set out with the right aims?
  - Did we have the right people?
  - Did the participants (and so, we) work well together?
  - Was the process of the meeting managed well enough?
  - Did the meeting achieve the set aims?

Points to Ponder

- Think back over some meetings that you have attended. What made the difference between a well-run and badly-run meeting?
- What about the next meeting that you have been asked to arrange or attend? What could you say or do either before or at the meeting that could make it a more useful experience?

Speaking up during a meeting, knowing what to say and getting your opinion across in an assertive manner can be daunting, particularly if more formal meetings are new to you. Sometimes, it can be useful to have a few phrases up your sleeve. You will of course have your own style and so not all of the phrases in Table 8.1 will feel comfortable (although they should provide a good starting point).

Table 8.1 General phrases to use in a meeting

What to say when you...	Suggested phrase
Want to give your view	'I've had some thoughts about this and...'
Want to interrupt	'I'd like to come in here'
Want to hear someone else's view	'Dan, how do you feel about/see this issue?'
Want to acknowledge (but not necessarily agree) with a comment	'Mmm' or 'That's an interesting point'
Agree with someone else's point	'I agree' or 'Yes, I feel that way too'
Disagree with someone else's point	'I have a different view on this' or 'I see this a bit differently'
You want to make a suggestion	'How about...' or 'I'd like to suggest that we...'
Consider that your comment has been ignored	'I'd just like to repeat...' or 'I just want to say again, that I don't...'
Feel that your comment has not been understood or has been misinterpreted	'Perhaps I need to explain myself differ-differently' or 'I just want to clarify a point'
Have not understood something	'I'm not quite sure I understand. Could you explain that last point again Mike'

Being asked to act as chairperson for a more formal meeting can be exciting and intimidating. Running a meeting means more than just working your way through the agenda. It is a skill (like others in this book) that can be learnt, practised and accomplished. Here are a few important points about the role.

- The chairperson is in charge of the process, stating and clarifying the aim of the meeting, guiding and facilitating discussions, managing problem-solving exercises and decision-making processes. Usually, the chair draws up the agenda and is responsible for arranging or delegating the setting up of the meeting and the writing up of the minutes.
- The role requires skills of communication, time-management, assertiveness, negotiation and delegation. Attitudes of firmness, calmness and confidence are essential. The key to successful 'chairing' is keeping control.
- It is the chairperson's responsibility to watch participants closely and to detect signs of lethargy, discouragement, confusion, stuckness, conflict, groupthink and scapegoating.

More specifically in the role of 'chair':

- start the meeting on time. It is quite common for a meeting not to start because 'Pauline' or 'Paulo' is not there yet. When meetings don't start on time, people think that they can arrive late as a matter of course and then it becomes the norm. Would you rush to get to a meeting on time when you knew that you would have to hang around for it to start?
- the agenda helps to guide and support the chairperson. Wherever possible, stick to it; it is the roadmap to your destination. If this is not possible make an explicit agreement to change it
- don't go through the minutes of the last meeting word by word. Hopefully they will have been circulated in time for people to have read them. Give people a couple of minutes just to remind themselves of the content
- it is your responsibility to encourage and to help people to discuss a point. If the discussion goes on for too long or does not seem to be going anywhere, you will have to intervene

- if a decision can't be made or a situation resolved, you may have to arrange to have another meeting or delegate someone to make the decision after the meeting
- arrange the date of the next meeting (if there is to be one) at the end of the current one. Trying to do it later is likely to be far more difficult
- unless it is absolutely impossible, end the meeting on time (or earlier). It is disrespectful and can be infuriating for a meeting to over-run (especially if it started late).

Tip

If this is your first time as the 'chair' you may wish to ask for feedback from a trusted participant afterwards.

If you are new to the role of chairperson and feel unsure about what to say in various situations, Table 8.2 lists a few useful phrases.

Table 8.2 Useful chairperson's phrases

What to say when...	Suggested phrase
Starting the meeting	'Good afternoon everyone and welcome. It's 2pm so let's make a start'
Welcoming guests	'I'd like to welcome Jean Brady to the meeting. Jean is the...'
Stating the aims of the meeting	'The aim of this meeting is to...'
Giving apologies for absence	'I have received apologies for absence from Derek who is unable to attend due to illness'
Referring to minutes of the last meeting	'Let's briefly go over the minutes of the meeting held on 6 January this year'
Asking for progress updates	'Fran, can you give us an update on the...'
Moving on to today's agenda	'Let's move on to today's agenda'
Establishing time boundaries	'We will finish promptly at 5pm'
Addressing the first agenda item	'So, the first agenda item is...'
Asking for input	'Would anyone like to add anything further?'
Drawing everything together	'Let's recap on the main points'
Closing an item and moving on to the next	'OK, thanks everyone. That covers that item. Let's move on to the next item on the agenda'
Asking for 'Any other Business'	'Would anyone like to raise any brief points under Any Other Business?'
Arranging the next meeting	'Let's set a date, time and location for the next meeting'
Thanking participants	'I'd like to thank you all for your input and work today and especially to Jean for her specialist contribution'
Ending the meeting	'It's 5pm and the meeting is closed'

Meetings can raise strong feelings in people and so the chairperson may have to handle difficult behaviour. Here are some common ways that people may behave during meetings and how to deal with them.

- *The late arrival* – 'Welcome Gill. We've just finished discussing holiday staffing issues. I'm sure that you can catch up in the tea break. We are now going to move on to discuss Bob's Health and Safety report. Bob, over to you.'
- *The person who hogs the limelight* – 'Thank you for your view Norman. What does everyone else think?'
- *The person who repeatedly interrupts* – 'Lori, I think, we'd all appreciate hearing what Mia has to say. Afterwards, we can hear your view.'
- *The person who is going round in circles* – 'Thank you, Lorraine. I'd just like to summarise the main points of your case.'
- *The silent participant* – 'Odi, I imagine that you've been reflecting on what has been said. I'm wondering what your view is on this?'
- *The person who leaves the meeting before the end* (and without due cause) – 'Valerie, I know that you are busy today. It's really important that we get your input on the staffing issue. Perhaps you could stay.'
- *The person who repeatedly talks to the chairperson instead of the participants* – 'What do we all think about Alan's point?'
- *The person who persistently wants to discuss a specific issue not on the agenda* – 'Thank you for raising this issue again Donald. I can see that this is important to you. As you know, it's not on the agenda for today's discussion so let's discuss it at a dedicated meeting.'
- *The person who tries to over-ride your decision that the meeting should end* – 'We've run out of time, Peter' or 'Peter, we'll have to leave that for another time. The meeting has ended.'

It's a Myth

Just because a person has not spoken during a meeting does not mean that they have not participated and contributed to the process.

In some settings, formal meetings may be inappropriate. However, it is important that people know what each is doing and how all of the tasks, roles and contributions fit together. One method is to hold a daily get-together that lasts for 5–10 minutes (depending on the number of people). Topics covered could include:

- what I achieved yesterday
- what I hope to achieve today
- what might be difficult
- what support might be welcome.

Who Said This?

Which famous American singer, born in 1958, said 'I live for meetings with men in suits. I love them because I know they've had a really boring week and I walk in there with my orange velvet leggings and drop popcorn in my cleavage and then fish it out and eat it. I like that. I know I'm entertaining them, and I know that they know':

(a) Chrissie Hynde?
(b) Madonna?
(c) Cyndi Lauper?

It's a Myth

Unless the purpose is to canvass as many views as possible, rarely do more participants make for a better meeting.

References

1 Adair J. *Effective Leadership*. London: Pan Books; 1988.
2 Tuckman BW. Development sequences in small groups. *Psycholog Bull*. 1965; **63**(6): 384–99.

Chapter 9

Speaking your mind and striking bargains

Giving and receiving feedback

If you criticize a mule, do it to his face.

Herbert V Prochnow

I can live for two months on a good compliment.

Mark Twain

'Come into my office will you. I've got some feedback on the way you handled that last project.' A neutral enough statement but oh..., the anxiety that can ensue!

Done correctly, the feedback process can have far-reaching and long-lasting positive results (constructive feedback). Done badly, as it often is, feedback can feel annihilating (destructive feedback).

But what is *feedback*? It's not the same as *criticism*, which is more about blame, making unfavourable or severe judgement. Nor is it the same as giving *compliments*, which are nice to give and nice to receive but in the end are just *nice*.

Feedback is well-considered, specific, accurate information, which is always designed to help the recipient.

Anyone can offer feedback to anyone else on any subject; it is not just the privilege of the manager. Feedback between colleagues and to your manager can help to build trust, respect and relationships.

We give feedback to:

- offer information that may expand a person's information about themselves
- provide information about the effect they have on others
- support or encourage desirable behaviour
- discourage undesirable behaviour
- help others to develop personally and professionally.

Tip

You may have heard the terms 'positive feedback' and 'negative feedback'; the former being about the good stuff that we do and the latter about the things that we could have done better. The problem is that when I hear 'negative feedback' I don't think 'Oh, good, I'm going to hear something difficult but I'm sure that it will be helpful to me'. No, I don't even get past the word 'negative'. To me, *all* feedback should in a sense be 'positive'; it should help the recipient to develop.

Most people have been on the receiving end of badly given, even destructive feedback. I know for myself the feelings of shame, guilt and anger that can result. Giving feedback well is an interpersonal skill that can be developed by acquiring knowledge, by experimentation and self-reflection.

Giving feedback

The feedback is likely to be more effective if you:

- give it face to face
- examine your motive for giving it. This should be with the aim of helping the other person, the patient, organisation, etc. (rather than helping you to feel superior, settle an old grudge or seek vengeance)
- give it near the time the behaviour has occurred (and before memories become cloudy). 'Why didn't somebody say something earlier? Then I could have had a chance to do something about it' is a sad phrase
- focus on the behaviour and not on the person as a whole
- give specific feedback, not generalisations, e.g. 'You were late three days this week' rather than 'You've been awfully late recently'
- talk about one thing at a time. Don't use it to criticise every wrongdoing the person has ever done. It can be very easy to get into 'While I've got you in here...' or 'And another thing...'
- give information about the consequences of the recipient's behaviour, e.g. 'When you don't do the filing each day, it mounts up on the desk and sometimes it falls on the floor. An important paper became lost this morning' rather than 'You are *so* disorganised'.
- give information about how you (or other people) feel in response to particular behaviours, e.g. 'When you shout like that, I feel afraid'
- own your own feelings, e.g. 'When you slammed the office door yesterday, I felt shocked' rather than 'When you slammed the office door yesterday, the staff felt shocked'
- give examples of what you have seen (or have been told by a reliable source has happened) not what you infer may have been happening. For example, 'At lunchtime, I heard you raise your voice to Maria. Would you be able to tell me about this?; sounds better than 'I heard you shouting at Maria. You don't like her do you?'
- know that the recipient can do something about their behaviour (otherwise, your feedback might feel like a punishment with no chance for the recipient to make things better)
- give information in the way that is best received by the recipient, avoiding words, terms, jargon, phrases or slang that the person is unlikely to understand
- use the 'feedback sandwich' technique. You say the bit that they may not want to hear in between two comments that you know they will like
- act in a sensitive way. Think about how the feedback may be received. Difficult feedback should be given in private
- don't press the person for an immediate response. This may be the first time that anyone has told them that they have been spotted picking their nose in public, so they may want time for it to sink in

- are prepared to listen (not throwing up your arms, walking off and saying 'I don't want to hear what excuses you have'). Use listening skills to show that you have understood (even if you don't agree). Don't get into a 'talk to the hand' scenario. If you don't listen to them, why should they listen to you?
- avoid exaggeration, e.g. 'You *always* get this wrong', and labelling, e.g. 'You really are so *lazy* you know'
- are aware of differences, including ability, age, gender, ethnic and religious background, sexual orientation and race.

Tip

Some people don't catch feedback the first time round and may benefit from the addition of written feedback.

It is important to follow feedback with a 'request for change'. How would you like the person to behave differently? In what way would this make a difference? What do they think about that request? They may have a better idea (or reject yours all together). Your feedback may of course be complimentary, in which case your request is that they continue (and perhaps develop) whatever it was they were doing.

'I praise loudly. I blame softly,' said Catherine the Great of Russia. Certainly, it is best to give difficult feedback in private. Being praised in front of colleagues can feel good and encourage others, but at other times, can lead to embarrassment for the recipient and envy and resentment among colleagues.

Tip

Try not to introduce your feedback with the commonplace phrase 'Don't take this the wrong way but…' or 'I'm not being personal but…'. We all know destructive feedback is on its way when we hear that 'but'.

Receiving feedback

Being able to *receive feedback* is a skill too. Many anticipate that feedback will be harsh, while others bat it away even when they know that it will be full of praise.

Here are some suggestions about how to receive feedback.

- Years ago, someone gave me some advice: 'Feedback? Breathe it in,' she said. I suppose what she meant was resist the temptation of 'blowing it away' by saying 'Oh, it was nothing' or 'I was just doing my job'.
- Listen carefully. Stay focused on hearing what is being said.
- Remember that you don't have to accept any of it (although you should listen).
- If you think that the feedback is too general, ask for more specific information.
- Ask questions that specify and clarify what is said. For example, 'Could you give an example of my sloppy timekeeping?' or 'When was the last time that I was late?'
- Acknowledge valid points.
- Take time to think about what has been said. If a response is necessary you

may wish to wait a while and to think through your response carefully. It is perfectly acceptable to say that you want to think over a situation and that you plan to get back to the other person in five minutes, tomorrow, next week, etc.

- Check that you have understood the feedback correctly by paraphrasing what has been said, e.g. 'So, what you are saying is that my time keeping hasn't been too good lately and if the situation doesn't improve, your next step will be to give me a verbal warning'.
- If the feedback is about an alleged incident that involved other people, ask them for their viewpoint.
- Remember that it may not have been easy for the other person to have given their feedback.

Afterwards, it's time to be honest with yourself. Try to remember the examples that have been given to you. Did you really behave in a particular way? Would other colleagues have given you the same feedback? Is this an isolated event or perhaps part of a pattern? Do you consider the feedback to have come from a person whose motive is honourable? Do you have a trusted colleague or friend who could tell you whether they agreed with all or part of the feedback.

Remember, you can accept some, all or none of the feedback.

Points to Ponder

- What has been your experience of receiving feedback? What have you learnt about this skill from times when feedback was delivered (a) well and (b) badly?
- Answer the following questions for an opportunity to assess your current use of feedback skills.

When giving feedback, do you…	*Yes*	*No*	*Not sure*
do it yourself rather than asking someone else to do it?			
usually give it face to face?			
always resist the temptation to get revenge on someone?			
for most of the time, use 'I' rather than 'We'?			
give specific examples?			
say how the recipient's behaviour is affecting people?			
resist the urge to drag bad stuff up from the past to add to your case?			
give it only when there is something that the recipient can do about it (either now or in future)?			
always try to use language that the recipient can understand?			
listen to the recipient's response?			
usually use the 'sandwich' method?			
make clear requests for change?			

- The more ticks in the 'Yes' column, the more effective you are likely to be at giving feedback. Areas that you may need to work on include those questions to which you answered 'No' or 'not sure'.

Experiment

Take another look at the questions to which you answered 'Not sure'. Over the next week or so, notice how you give feedback (particularly in relation to these areas). This can be at home (perhaps commenting on a domestic task carried out by a family member) or elsewhere.

Who Said This?

Which American actress, famous for her double entendres, said: 'It is better to be looked over than overlooked':

(a) Marilyn Monroe?
(b) Lucille Ball?
(c) Mae West?

Negotiating skills

The go-between wears many sandals.

Japanese proverb

Give me what I want. NOW!

A 6-year-old

On television and in the press, we hear a lot about the big negotiation scenarios – efforts to broker a deal between two warring countries, prevent industrial action or negotiate the release of a hostage.

Negotiation means 'to communicate with others in order to achieve an agreement'; in other words to 'bargain', 'haggle' or 'strike a deal'. For a situation to be negotiated there must be two or more people, groups or organisations who each want different outcomes but are all prepared to compromise and work towards a mutually acceptable outcome. The main point to remember about negotiation is that all sides want to resolve the situation.

Being able to negotiate well is a great interpersonal skill both at work and in the wider world. It saves time, reduces stress and improves relationships. Negotiation is a 'game' that is played well when both know the rules and are prepared to play by them. Around the negotiating table, good negotiators can be ruthless and fierce but away from it they may be the best of friends.

Negotiation:

• is not the same as persuasion (although there may be elements of persuasion in the process)
• ideally, should never involve manipulation but does require you to know how to 'play the game'
• is about achieving a win/win result. A win/lose result is, in effect, the same as lose/lose. You may have won in the short term but it is unlikely that any agreed action will be followed up or performed well. The loser is likely to approach future negotiations with a 'win at all costs' attitude.

Point to Ponder

Does a 'win/win' result feel possible to you?

Negotiation can only happen when:

- there is disagreement
- both parties are willing to reach an agreement (if at all possible)
- each party has available assets and the authority to trade them.

Sometimes, negotiation is not the best way forward. *Don't negotiate when*:

- the subject is non-negotiable, e.g. the safety of a patient
- the other person is in total agreement with you. Some people just love to haggle
- one person or party does not want to negotiate. Both must (in principle) be prepared to go through the process
- you have no authority to negotiate, e.g. you are not the decision maker
- you have nothing to trade.

Points to Ponder

- Are you a good negotiator or do you have the makings of one? Look at the 10 attitudes listed below. Can you lay claim to some?

Attitude	*Yes*	*No*	*Don't know*
Have a good level of self-understanding.			
Believe that people can reach a win/win outcome			
Have a willingness to explore the other person's position			
Have a wish to understand the other person's position			
Can act confidently and assertively			
Only promise what you can deliver			
Usually know the facts to back up your case			
Be willing to give things away (but only if you get something in return)			
Perseverance			
Honesty			

- How many attitudes were you able to identify? Would you benefit from developing any? How could you go about doing that?

All negotiation requires some degree of preparation; the higher the stakes, the more preparation needed. Asking yourself the following questions may help you to prepare effectively.

1 What do you know about the other person (let's call him 'Andy') and his situation?
2 Think about the relationship – is it a new one? Have you negotiated with Andy before? How did it go? What is his style?
3 What common ground do you have? What can you build upon?
4 What do you want to get out of this negotiation?

5   What do you think Andy wants to get out of it?
6   What would be a realistic outcome for you?
7   What do you imagine would be a realistic outcome for Andy?
8   Apart from what Andy has told you he wants, what else might interest him, i.e. what else could you use as a 'bargaining chip'?
9   What are you prepared to lose?
10 What must you keep at all costs?
11 What do you imagine Andy would be prepared to lose?
12 What do you imagine Andy will want to keep at all costs?
13 Does a deal have to be reached or can you afford to walk away? Can Andy?

Some important rules to remember when preparing to negotiate.

1 There is usually a better deal to be had but you must make a proposal.
2 Never give anything away without getting something back. Everything has a value.
3 Propose changes rather than complaining about the current situation.
4 Acknowledge any forward movement and concessions made by the other person.
5 Be specific about details, e.g. times, places, people. Especially make sure that you do this near the end of a long negotiating process when sheer relief mixed with tiredness may lull you into a false sense of completion.
6 Document all decisions.
7 If you get what you want (or most of what you want) resist the temptation to revel in it, especially in front of the other person.
8 If you are not successful, don't sulk. Go for a cup of tea and think how you might do it differently the next time you negotiate.

Tip

Remember that cultures respond to and approach the negotiating process in different ways. Keep an eye out for cultural stereotypes.

It is important to get the physical environment right before you begin to negotiate. Unless absolutely unavoidable or advantageous to you, try to meet on neutral territory. Don't sit around a table unless you have a lot of paperwork, in which case try to get a round table. If this is not possible, sit 'around the corner' to each other. If, for each negotiating position, there is more than one person, intersperse everyone. Attention to this type of detail encourages collaboration and a culture of 'we' rather than 'them versus us'.

Use active listening skills to explore the other person's position. Open questions enable you to find out about the other person's position. Reflecting, paraphrasing and summarising helps you to track progress, keeps the discussion on track, stops people going round in circles and helps clear up any small misunderstandings. Silence gives you time to think. Empathy helps you to understand and communicate that understanding of the other person's position. A genuineness will help other people to trust you, and while you will have to make judgements about offers made, a non-judgemental attitude towards the other person will help the process. Jargon-free language can help to prevent feelings of disempowerment. Promote good feeling by using phrases such as

'We're making good progress' or 'We are on the way to an agreement'. End the negotiation process in a good way with an acknowledgement of the work done and concessions made by both sides.

Sometimes, the negotiating process reaches 'deadlock'. This is not the same as lose/lose or an end to the negotiation process. It is merely a suspension of the process and does mean that both sides still have faith that the process could work (otherwise they would have walked away). It's like being halfway across a bridge; you could turn around and go all the way back to the start, but with a little extra push you might just make it to the other side. You must keep exploring, to find that *one* thing that will allow you both to recommence negotiations. Offer one small thing – it may be all that is needed to get things moving again. If this doesn't work, take a short break, come back to the negotiating table and restate your position. Yours may not have changed, but theirs might have done. If after this you still face deadlock, set an agreed deadline (it may help to focus you both). If this doesn't work, it may be wise to change negotiators or call in a mediator.

Like any 'game', negotiation has its own 'dirty tricks'. People use them because (a) their job depends upon success 'at all costs', (b) the idea of not getting what they want is unbearable or (c) they don't care about the current or future relationship with the other negotiator.

I want to give you some information about some of these dirty tricks. My hope is that you will use it to spot and understand these behaviours. In this way, you can lessen their impact. I don't recommend their use to those who want to negotiate in an ethical way. While there are many more, Table 9.1 lists a selection that I have called 'The Dirty Dozen'.

Points to Ponder

- Have you (a) ever used or (b) been on the receiving end of any of these 'dirty tricks'. Were there any short- or longer-term consequences?
- Pick three tactics from the 'Dirty Dozen'. If, in the middle of negotiations, someone tried to use these tactics, how might you respond (a) if you could say anything and (b) if you had to give a more considered response?

Dirty trick #1...

My response (if I could say anything)...

My considered response...

Dirty trick #2...

My response (if I could say anything)...

My considered response...

Dirty trick #3...

My response (if I could say anything)...

My considered response...

Table 9.1 The Dirty Dozen

Tactic	What may be going on and what to do about it
'Let's meet in my office'	Seeking territorial advantage. Meet on neutral ground
'If you don't agree, there's no point in me staying'	Threat. Say that you want to meet with someone who can negotiate. You could call their bluff and agree to end the meeting
'As I see it, we have two options available'	Both of which are theirs. Usually, there are more options for consideration (yours, for example)
'Look. I'm going to be straight here'	Perhaps you need to check out with them that they have been straight with you so far.
'We only have 10 more minutes to get this sorted out'	Schedule another meeting
'I'm not sure that your colleagues agree with you'	Divide and conquer tactic
'I'll have to defer that decision to my manager and that will take more time'	As they clearly have no decision-making power, say that you want to end this meeting and talk to their manager yourself
'I'll be in trouble if I don't get your agreement on this'	That is not your responsibility. Suggest that they discuss the 'oppressive regime' that they appear to be under with their manager
'It has been decided'	So why are we having this meeting?
'Look, I've been reasonable so far'	Good. Long may it continue
'Look, my colleague here doesn't think that I should accept your offer but I'd really like to tie things up with you'	We've all seen the Good Cop/Bad Cop scenarios in Police dramas. Don't be drawn in
'Do you really have the authority to make this decision?'	Attempt to undermine you. They know that you are the decision-maker otherwise they would be talking to someone else

---

Tip

Some people 'flinch' when an offer is made that they don't want to accept. I wouldn't go so far as to describe it as a 'dirty trick', but it can be manipulative. The flinch may be a genuine reaction, but if you are pretty certain that it was for your benefit, coolly say 'You look a bit shocked. I'm wondering what you were expecting me to say?'. That way you get them to talk about their unrealistic expectations rather than what they consider to be your 'ridiculous' offer.

Point to Ponder

Remember a time when you lost out because you could have negotiated a better deal. What stopped you? If the situation presented itself again, what might you do differently?

Who Said This?

Which famous British prime minister and author said 'Better to jaw-jaw than to war-war':

(a) Winston Churchill?
(b) Harold Wilson?
(c) Tony Blair?

Part IV: Taking care of yourself

Chapter 10

Emotional wellbeing

Stress – the good, the bad and the ugly

Health is a state of complete physical, mental and social well-being and not merely the absence of disease or infirmity.

World Health Organization[1]

When a person has emotional and mental wellbeing, they not only feel freedom from distress but can:

- have fun and engage in adult play
- be creative
- express feelings and thoughts as appropriate
- feel 'good enough'
- be confident and assertive
- find, develop and maintain healthy relationships
- enjoy both solitude and company
- show care and concern for self and for others
- ask for help without feeling a failure
- tackle problems, solve them and learn from them
- have a sense of connectedness and belonging
- contribute to society
- be aware of what really matters in life.

Points to Ponder

- How many signs of emotional and mental wellbeing can you identify at the moment?
- Which would you like to develop more and how might you do that?

Wouldn't it be great to be able to put our hand up to all of these signs? Alas, it is a rare person who can do this; for most, 'a stressful life' gets in the way. But what do I mean by 'stressful'?

We talk about 'stress' as if it were always a bad thing to be avoided at all costs, but in fact, there are two types of 'stress'.

1 Eustress – the 'feeling the pressure'; a sense of excitement and challenge. When a task has these qualities we feel galvanised into action and enthusiastic. Overcoming little challenges makes life more satisfying. Too little excitement and stimulation can lead to boredom and apathy. We all need a certain amount of eustress in our life.

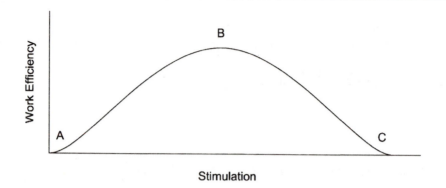

Figure 10.1 The effect of stimulation on work efficiency.

2 Distress – happens when that pressure and stimulation continues for a long time without opportunity for the person to recover. We become like an elastic band, stretched and stretched until eventually, it snaps. This is what people call 'stress'.

For some people, 'stress' has become a buzz word. What they mean is that they are a little bit more busy than usual. But for others, stress is a real problem that affects their life, work and relationships.

Figure 10.1. illustrates the relationship between stimulation and efficiency at work. Too little stimulation leads to low efficiency (A). Too much stimulation also leads to low efficiency and, in addition, collapse (C). Just the right amount of stimulation leads to efficiency at work (B).

When eustress becomes distress, ability to care effectively for ourselves and others is affected, morale falls, absenteeism goes up and staff retention goes down. More mistakes occur, co-workers become involved in conflict and there is less time for patients, relatives and carers.

Employees begin to disempower themselves by placing control and responsibility outside of themselves and onto 'the system'. We say, 'I can't do anything about it. It's just the way it is' and we joke by saying 'Don't ask me, I only work here'.

Point to Ponder

What is your experience of being stretched and stimulated in a eustress type of way?

Did You Know?

In 2004/05, 12.8 million working days were lost to stress, depression and anxiety.[2]

'Stress' has been defined in various ways.

• 'Stress arises when individuals perceive that they cannot adequately cope with the demands being made on them or with threats to their well-being.'[3]

- 'Stress is the psychological, physiological and behavioural response by an individual when they perceive a lack of equilibrium between the demands placed upon them and their ability to meet those demands, which, over a period of time, leads to ill-health.'[4]

In other words, stress occurs when what we are asked to do is greater than what we perceive as our ability to cope. Note the word 'perceive', which means that it need not be based on reality. The demands mentioned can be external (e.g. deadlines, relationships, financial) or internal (e.g. beliefs, habits, thoughts, imaginings). Often, it is the internal demands that cause us more problems than the external ones (but more about this later).

In many ways, and with all our technological advances, humans have come a long way. But not as far as stress is concerned. The problem is that the part of the brain that, during prehistoric times, protected primitive men and women from daily dangers of sabre-toothed tigers and marauding tribes has not developed much since that time. Now, when we perceive ourselves to be 'under attack' from conflicting pressures, difficult relationships, etc., our brain still acts as if these things were life-threatening. It does not see these modern-day 'tigers' as relatively safe, but launches into a decision. Do I fight (and possibly win), take flight, run (and maybe escape) or stay still (and act dead)?

Part of being able to manage stress is the ability to understand what is going on, to make sense of it and the strange things that happen to the body, mind and behaviour during the 'crisis'. Let's take a very common symptom of stress – diarrhoea. It doesn't make sense. Rushing to the toilet isn't going to resolve the fact that my boss is bullying me or that I have growing financial debt. But to have diarrhoea makes perfect sense to that primitive part of our brain. I stand a better chance of not ending up as a sabre-toothed tiger's dinner if I can run faster. One way to do this is to make myself lighter by losing the contents of my guts. As an added bonus to me, animals don't like their food to be contaminated by faeces and so I might just escape. Now it makes sense. Most of the worrying things that happen when stressed can be explained as part of a self-protective mechanism; actually our bodies are functioning extremely well.

What are our 'modern-day tigers'? The Social Readjustment Rating Scale proposes the degree of readjustment required following a life event. Holmes and Rahe made a link between life events and illness. In the two years preceding an illness, 300 or more Life Change Units worth of stressful events had occurred.[5] What is interesting is that while many of these 'life events' are generally considered unpleasant, some are usually regarded as pleasant, e.g. marriage and Christmas. Conducted in the 1960s, the study reflects the social culture of that time but is still valid today. Table 10.1 lists some of the life events and their effect.

Case study

During the past two years, Mandy and her husband separated mainly because their sex life was non-existent. They went to couples counselling and got their sex life back on track and began to live together again. Having got back together, Mandy became pregnant. With a 4-year-old son and a new baby about to be born, they moved to a larger house. Their son started school, the new baby was born and Mandy was feeding him three times a night. Later that year they all went on holiday together.

Table 10.1 Effect of life events

Life events	Life Change Units
Minor violation of the law	11
Christmas	12
Holiday	13
Change in eating habits	15
Change in sleeping patterns	16
Change in recreation patterns	19
Change in residence	20
Child begins school	26
Taking on a large mortgage	31
Gain of a new family member	39
Sexual difficulty	39
Pregnancy	40
Marital reconciliation	45
Death of close family member	63
Marital separation	65
Death of spouse	100

Not an unusual story but Mandy scored enough points to put her at increased risk of illness.

But what about work-related stress? Holmes and Rahe found that they could apply their theory to this area too (Table 10.2).

Here are some other work-related stressors. Sometimes there is *not enough*:

- stimulating and varied work that has meaning and significance
- appreciation shown by colleagues, management and users of the service
- trust and faith from colleagues, managers, patients
- control, scope for use of initiative and consultation
- clear and supportive communication
- supervision and support for development, e.g. training and promotion
- acknowledgement that dealing with 'the public', ill, dying or distressed can be stressful
- emphasis put on good co-worker relationships
- up-to-date and working technology
- flexible work schedules
- attention paid to creating a pleasant work environment.

Table 10.2 Effect of work-related life events

Life events	Life Change Units
Change in work conditions or hours	20
Trouble with boss	23
Change in responsibility at work	29
Change to a different line of work	36
Change in financial state	38
Business readjustment	39
Retirement	45
Getting the sack	47

There may be *too much*:

- work with unrealistic deadlines
- collusion with long hours culture
- imposed work/life imbalance
- role confusion or conflict
- staff turnover and absenteeism
- unsupported change and restructuring
- too much new technology to learn about
- risk of physical and emotional abuse, including bullying, harassment and discrimination
- blame
- being at the mercy of changing political policy.

Points to Ponder

- How many of these work-related stressors can you identify?
- What changes could you make to reduce some of these things? For example, consider your physical environment, what simple change could you make today that would make it feel a little better?

The ability to cope with and bounce back from stressful events and continuing stressors depends on how much *resilience* we have. I'm sure you know of some people who, although hit by illness, tragedy, etc., after a while were able to recover, while others never seemed to get back on their feet. In part, resilience develops through being confronted with and successfully tackling stressful events and situations. Being resilient is not the same as being 'hard', 'uncaring' or 'insensitive', but means being able to rely and depend upon yourself. It is not the same as 'fierce independence', because a resilient person can ask others for help when necessary. A resilient person shows three specific character traits.

1 A sense of commitment – an involvement and sense of purpose.
2 A feeling of being in control – a belief that they have some control in a difficult situation.
3 Challenge – a sense of being open to new experiences.

Point to Ponder

How resilient do you see yourself as being? What would other people say about you?

You can build up your resilience levels by using the following two strategies together.

1 Reassuring self-talk, e.g. 'I will be OK. I've been through this situation before and I survived then. I can get through this' or 'I have lots of friends who could help me if necessary'.
2 Facing up to and confronting yourself, e.g. 'OK. What do I need to develop within myself to be able to handle this situation? Perhaps I could be more assertive'.

It is important that you practise *both* components. If all you do is calm and reassure yourself without confronting you end up feeling a nice warm feeling but you don't get any further than that, whereas if all you do is confront yourself you end up feeling battered and bruised.

Points to Ponder

- Think of a difficult situation that you have been in? How did you cope?
- What reassurance (if any) did you give yourself? How did you confront yourself (if at all)?
- Do you find it easier to reassure or confront yourself? How could you address any imbalance?

While a short-lived episode of stress is unlikely to harm a person, chronic stress has been linked to various illnesses, e.g. digestive problems, bladder disturbances, chronic insomnia, some cancers, diabetes, rheumatoid arthritis, asthma, high blood pressure, stroke, coronary problems, sexual problems, susceptibility to some infections, back pain, depression, anxiety and substance abuse.

Another consequence of prolonged stress is 'burnout'. Previously thought to be confined to executives, burnout is common among the helping professions and is a state of physical, mental, emotional and spiritual exhaustion. When a person is burnt out, they have lost their resilience (the ability to take a knock and bounce back). There is sense of disenchantment of what previously was valued. It is the body and mind's way of saying 'Enough!'

When a person suffers burnout three signs present together.

1 Feelings of being emotionally overstretched, worn out by work and contact with other people (particularly those to whom the service is offered).
2 A negative, cold and impersonal response towards these people.
3 An absence of feelings of competence and successful achievement at work.

(Maslach and Jackson, 1981).[6]

Point to Ponder

Do you identify with any of these three signs? Do you have all three?

Some ways to prevent burnout include:

- setting limits and boundaries in life. Learning to say 'No'
- bringing variety into your life
- deciding and focusing on priorities and life goals
- reviewing work/life balance (see later)
- practising time management
- becoming 'stress aware'
- practising relaxation
- sleeping, eating and exercising well (see later)
- giving yourself positive affirmation
- looking for activities and things that give your life meaning and significance
- making and maintaining relationships that have a balance of give and take
- finding new projects to initiate, e.g. a hobby
- remembering that you are 'only human' with limits.

Points to Ponder

- How much do you consider yourself to be at risk of burnout?
- What steps could you put in place to reduce your chances of burnout?
- If you were to burn out, what would you do? Who could help you?

If you are concerned about stress or burnout, talk to your GP or occupational health department.

Did You Know?

About half a million people in the UK experience work-related stress at a level they believe is making them ill. Up to 5 million people in the UK feel 'very' or 'extremely' stressed by their work.[2]

Who Said This?

Which famous American boxer refused to serve in the army during the Vietnam War and said: 'It's just a job. Grass grows, birds fly, waves pound the sand. I beat people up':

(a) Joe Frazier?
(b) Muhammad Ali?
(c) George Foreman?

Recognising stress

> *Stress is an ignorant state. It believes that everything is an emergency.*
> Natalie Goldberg[7]

No one suddenly becomes 'stressed'; the problem with stress is that it creeps up on people. To be able to manage stress in our lives it is important to recognise the early signs along the way.

Signs of stress can be divided into how it affects five aspects of us.

1 Our physical being.
2 Our emotional being.
3 Our thinking.
4 Our behaviour.
5 Our spiritual or philosophical outlook.

How many of these *physical* signs of stress have you experienced in the past month?

- Changes to heartbeat, chest tightness, breathlessness, feeling faint.
- Digestive changes – constipation, indigestion, increased visits to toilet (diarrhoea and urination), nausea and vomiting.
- Dry mouth, headaches, aching limbs, shaking.
- Skin complaints that arise or worsen, hot and cold sweats.

- Feeling overly tired (without apparent reason).
- Increased sensitivity to pain.

How many *emotional* signs of stress have you experienced in the last month?

- Anxiety, irritability, anger, over-reaction to situations.
- Feeling low or sad (without apparent reason).
- Feeling guilty, ashamed, unjustified jealousy.
- Feeling emotionless.

How many of these types of *thoughts* have you experienced in the past month?

- 'Everyone is against me.'
- 'No one cares about me.'
- 'I don't care any more.'
- 'I'm a failure.'
- 'I have no control over my life.'
- 'It's like I've gone blank.'
- 'I can't think straight.'
- 'My worries just keep going round and round in my head.

Let's look at the *behavioural* signs of stress. How many have you experienced in the past month?

- Change in use of substances (alcohol, smoking, caffeine, drugs, self-medication), eating habits (over, under, craving).
- Decreased desire to go to work or to do usual activities and hobbies.
- Increase in relationship problems, conflict, wanting to isolate and not socialise, changes in sexual desire and activity.
- Obsessive behaviour, e.g. checking rituals, phobias (that worsen or arise).
- Suicidal or self-harming behaviour.
- Insomnia.
- Crying.
- Teeth grinding.

Stress can also affect our *spiritual* and *philosophical* outlook on life. Have you had any of these types of concerns in the past month?

- Life has no meaning any more.
- A sense of disconnection from what is important.
- A lingering sense of unease.
- A lack of perspective.

A Word of Caution

Most people will, at some time, have a few of these stress indicators; they are part of being alive. It is the number of indicators happening at any one time and their frequency coupled with how bad they are, that is important. If you are concerned about any of these indicators or if they are affecting your life, discuss them with your GP. They can help you to deal with your stress levels (more about this later) but can also check that they are not due to an underlying medical condition, e.g. thyroid disease, depression, diabetes.

Did You Know?

'Bruxism' (grinding of teeth) generates a force large enough to crack a walnut (and your teeth). It is a common occurrence during periods of stress.

It's a Myth

'Minor' indicators of stress, such as indigestion or headache, should not be ignored. These are important early warning signs that something is not right and requires attention.

How our thoughts influence our emotional wellbeing

People are disturbed not by things but by the views which they take of them.

Epictetus

As early as 100 BC, links were beginning to be made between what we think and how we feel.

In an earlier section, we looked at the demands that may be placed on you from the outside. Now, it's time to look at the tricky subject of how we make demands upon ourselves. These inner demands usually stem from messages received while growing up. Many childhood messages were useful to us, e.g. 'It's good to tell the truth'. Although they helped shape us into worthwhile people, these messages carried implications, e.g. 'People should (and will) be honest with me'. We grow up with expectations of how people (and ourselves) 'should' be. Another common message that we tell ourselves is 'I must work hard (or else)'. When these beliefs conflict with the realities of life, stress can result.

The first step towards understanding, questioning and possibly changing these messages is to notice them.

Points to Ponder

- Off the top of your head and without applying too much thought or judgement, finish off these sentence stems about how you and other people should behave: e.g. 'I must put other people's needs before mine' or 'People should never let me down.'
  - I/Other people should...
  - I/Other people must...
  - I/Other people ought...
- As you make these demands inside your head notice how you feel.
- Now, change the statements to begin with 'I would prefer to...' or 'I would rather people...'
- Notice any difference in how that feels.
- Are the messages about how you or other people should/must/ought to behave realistic today? Now that as an adult you have a greater appreciation of the grim realities of life, could you modify or get rid of any of these messages?

Most people have a well-developed habit of distorting otherwise perfectly rational thoughts. Here are 10 very common ways that we do it.

- *Overgeneralisation* – applying a general rule to all situations or people, e.g. 'Of course, all of the people in that department are late for work every day.'
- *Magnification* – events become catastrophes, e.g. 'My girlfriend has just dumped me. I'll never, ever find anyone else.'
- *Minimisation* – a denial of how serious things are, e.g. 'I know I've got a stomach ulcer but it's only a little one. I can eat and drink whatever I want.'
- *Personalisation* – relating events to self and taking things too personally, e.g. 'My boss looks angry today. I expect that's my fault.'
- *Dichotomous thinking* – black-and-white thinking, e.g. 'If I don't get this absolutely right, I'm a total failure.'
- *Tunnel vision* – seeing only one part of the picture, a narrow-mindedness, e.g. 'I only ever wear black clothes.'
- *Negative labelling* – attaching labels to people then seeing them as that label, e.g. 'These days, all adolescents are delinquents. Look there goes another one of them!'
- *Mind reading* – the idea that you can read the minds of other people and that they should be able to read yours, e.g. 'I know she doesn't like me. We've never spoken but I just know that she doesn't' or 'He should have known that I wouldn't like that idea.'
- *Subjective reasoning* – the belief that if I feel an emotion strongly enough then it must be justified, e.g. 'I *feel* guilty therefore I *am* guilty.'
- *Perfectionism*, e.g. 'I got 98% for my latest assignment. I'm going to go over it and see where I lost that 2%.'

Point to Ponder

Do any of these mechanisms sound familiar?

Given that most of us have internal messages and distorted thoughts, apart from becoming aware of them, what else can we do? Socrates, the ancient Greek philosopher, devised a selection of questions aimed at finding evidence to dispute thoughts that upset us and may be distorted. The sort of *Socratic Questions* that you could ask yourself include the following.

- What's the evidence for this?
- Who says that this must be the case?
- What is the worst thing that could happen? And if it did, what then?
- Is there another way of looking at this?
- Is there any other explanation for this?
- What are the advantages of maintaining this view?
- What are the disadvantages of maintaining this view?
- What would a friend say about my situation?

If you absolutely *must* use your own thoughts to stress yourself, remember these *Ten Rules for Living Stressfully*.

1 I must be nice (at all times).

2 Others must like me (or else I will feel awful).
3 If I say that I'll do something, I must do it at all costs.
4 I should put others before myself.
5 I should be able to do anything (and without help).
6 I must never be late (for anything).
7 I must never make a mistake.
8 I must never let anyone down.
9 I must never feel upset.
10 Being human is not an option.

Did You Know?

While a positive mental attitude can be very helpful in preventing stress, some people go a bit far. 'Pollyannaism' is another example of distorted thinking whereby there exists a tendency to be over-optimistic, even in the face of great adversity. The term is derived from a children's book, written in 1913 by EH Porter.[8] *Pollyanna* tells the story of a girl, adopted by her aunt and taken to live in a miserable and despondent town. After a while in Pollyanna's infectious, 'cheery' company, the town's inhabitants also became very happy. While the book was never meant to suggest a belittling of the 'positive mental attitude', the term 'Pollyannaism' has become part of psychological terminology.

What can I do to help myself?

If it is to be. It is up to me.

William H Johnson

Self-help strategies can be divided into two types, those that:

- offer short-term fixes
- help to reduce or prevent the occurrence of stress-related symptoms.

The short-term fixes or palliative approaches, work quickly and require little effort. As with most things in life, these strategies have a downside. Before we look at these, I want to tell you about 'Anita', a stressed-out receptionist, working in an Accident and Emergency department in an inner city.

Case study

Anita was just about coping with a very stressful and longstanding situation at work. There had been big changes in her role and her shift pattern. Let's consider some of the strategies that Anita used to get by (as well as some that she rejected).

  Anita was really fed up. At work, nothing seemed the same any more. There had been such big changes in the department and in the restructuring, she had lost colleagues who, over the years, had become friends. Worse still, they had been replaced by people that she had to train up. At the same time, she was expected to learn 'the ropes' of her new job. Anita's boss was on her back because the department wasn't reaching its targets and when she tried to talk to him, he just raised his hand and said 'I know… we're all in the same boat, Anita.' Becoming increasingly dissatisfied with having to wait longer, the patients were complaining and so were blaming Anita.

In an effort to keep up, she began to take paperwork home. While her family knew that she was under pressure, they were beginning to feel neglected.

Anita was having problems sleeping. Often, a glass of wine would help to relax her and she and her husband started to enjoy wine with their evening meal. One day, instead of a bottle, Anita bought a wine box (it was better value after all). But it also meant that she began to drink more. She woke up with headaches and had begun to develop backache (something that she had never suffered from before).

She bought some codeine tablets, which gave some welcome relief at first, but after a while Anita had to increase the dose. Soon, she was taking more than the recommended dose. She wondered whether the pharmacist might notice and so was buying the tablets from different pharmacies (just in case).

At least, now she was falling asleep at night (although she was waking up in the middle of the night and finding it difficult to go back to sleep). Anita began to feel 'spaced out' during the day and took up drinking coffee again (something she had given up a few years ago).

Her husband suggested that they have a night out with friends but she was just too tired. Anyway, she had begun to feel bored and disinterested in their friends. Anita knew that she could always rely on her wine box and her codeine. They would never let her down.

Clearly Anita was suffering from workplace stress and this was beginning to impact on her life at home and her health. The strategies that she had put in place worked in the short term, but after a while became problems in themselves. Anita's way of coping is not unusual; she dealt with it the best way that she knew how.

Let's look at a couple of the self-help approaches that Anita used.

- There is growing evidence that small amounts of alcohol can improve your health. Wine, beer, a gin and tonic perhaps, are a very quick way of 'stepping out of yourself' for a while and may be just what is needed to de-stress you at the end of a difficult day. The problem is that alcohol is an addictive substance to which a tolerance can easily build up, leading to more drinking. We are very good at fooling ourselves when it comes to drinking. Some people say: 'I never drink alone' (but may go to the pub every night with friends and drink three double gins). Many people who have a dependency on alcohol convince themselves that they could 'stop tomorrow', but most never do.
- Anita has become dependent on codeine, easily available from any pharmacy. The developed world has a growing problem with dependency on over-the-counter (OTC) medication. Codeine-based painkillers and cough mixtures containing alcohol seem to be the most commonly over-used OTC medicines.

Anita's symptoms of stress were not pleasant and whilst it is understandable that she wanted to get rid of them, perhaps she could have regarded them as a message.

The positive aspects of the 'short-term fix' are that most are readily available and act quickly. The downside is that they don't address the underlying problem. You may have to take more and more to get the same effect and some may cause you more harm than whatever was stressing you in the first place.

Point to Ponder

Do you use any of Anita's quick-fix strategies when you feel stressed? Perhaps you have others? How have they helped? Have they had any other consequences?

There are many different ways to prevent and tackle stress that will not harm you. These strategies require you to invest some effort and may have financial implications. The amount of effort and the amount of money needed will depend on which one(s) you choose.

Work/life balance

As my life progresses, the more I find the word 'balance' gaining relevance and significance. The term 'work/life balance' itself suggests an interesting split – there is 'work' and then there is 'everything else'. Now, I know what job I do, when I do it, where I do it and (usually) what I will be required to do, but what is involved in the 'everything else'? I could define it as 'the things I do when I'm not at work'. That feels too general for me to make informed choices about my 'life', let alone decide whether there is an imbalance. Work/life balance is all about spreading our time, energy, resources and effort in a way that helps to keep us healthy.

What happens when there is an imbalance? Life becomes unsteady and we lose our composure. Imagine a tightrope walker who is perfectly safe as long as they keep their balance. But what happens when a lion roars and they start to wobble? If they can regain their balance then they will be OK, if not, they will fall.

One way to look at how balanced your life is, is to divide your time up like a pie (Figure 10.2). Each slice represents a part of your life, e.g. family, home,

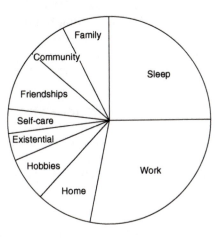

Figure 10.2 Life's activities.

friendships, community, hobbies, self-care, existential (religious/spiritual/philosophical concerns/questions about life) and, of course, work.

Experiment

Try drawing your life activity pie. There are 168 hours in a week. Work out how much time you spend sleeping and mark that in. Now put in time spent working (including travel time). Then divide the remaining time between the other activities. What does *your* pie look like? How would you like it to look? What changes would you need to make in order to achieve this?

Tip

Instead of looking at your work/life balance in terms of time, you could repeat the exercise this time estimating how much interest, energy, enthusiasm or commitment you put into each area.

Stress diary

A stress diary is more than just a list of stressful events that happened today. It is a good way of finding out what types of things stress you, who might be stressing you, when and how you respond to stressors and the strategies that you use. Taking stock at the end of each day can help you to wind down. If you do this for two to three weeks, you should begin to see patterns emerge. You will gain some understanding of what stress level feels comfortable (and stimulating) for you and what begins to make you want to tear your hair out.

Social support

You may remember that Anita didn't want to socialise. During times of stress, it is a very common response to want to tell friends and family that you 'can't be bothered' or 'feel too tired' when they suggest a get-together or night out. You may well feel exhausted by what is happening to you, but unless these people are the *cause* of your stress, you would be wise to accept their offer. Social support is the physical and emotional comfort and succour given to us by family, friends, colleagues and people in our community. Support from people can come in various forms. For example:

• listening to each other's problems, showing concern, phoning someone just to say: 'You know that I'm here if you need me'
• showing an understanding through experience, e.g. offering viewpoints, opinions and suggestions that might help
• day-to-day help, e.g. looking after a friend's baby so that she can catch up on some sleep.

When people come for counselling, I often ask: 'What social support do you have?' Sometimes, helping a person to identify potential sources can preclude the need for further counselling.

> **Point to Ponder**
>
> Who are your 'social supporters' (both in and out of work)?

Diet

Although a very controversial area, there is evidence that food choices may have some effect on serotonin levels, the neurotransmitter that improves mood and helps us to cope better with stress. Apart from the actual chemical components in food, most people feel better after having had a meal prepared with thought and care, compared to something just 'thrown together'. When stressed, it is incredibly easy to raid the fridge and snack on 'sugar-rush' foods. Motivation to keep at a healthy weight falls and we experience reduced appetite for healthy food. When busy, the opportunities to be able to think about, choose, buy, cook and eat healthy food may be reduced. We can easily fall into a vicious circle.

> **Point to Ponder**
>
> When we tell ourselves that we are too busy to eat properly – what message are we sending ourselves?

Sleep

How well did you sleep last night? Prolonged periods of sleeplessness may result from a stressful life or can be the cause of it. Tiredness, difficulty in being able to concentrate and make decisions, headaches, feeling nauseous and emotionally low are just some of the effects of insomnia.

How much sleep do you need? It all depends on how old you are. A child may need 9–10 hours a night while most adults need 7–8 hours. A few people seem to be able to get by with very little sleep.

A stressful existence can make it difficult for you to fall asleep and/or stay asleep. Even if you do stay asleep, stress can lead to anxiety dreams and other sleep disturbances.

Here are a few tips for getting a good night's sleep.

- Establish and maintain a regular bedtime routine; if the brain knows what to expect, it will begin to wind down. Develop a 'going-to-bed' ritual.
- Don't eat too late and limit your caffeine and alcohol intake. Alcohol gets you to sleep but can make you wake up in the middle of the night. It can also make you more prone to snoring (which may not be a problem to you, but can be hellish for those lying next to you).
- If you are not asleep after 20–25 minutes, get up and do something boring (or perhaps boring and useful, like the ironing). After 30 minutes, go back to bed. As we all know from attending tedious meetings, a bored brain is a sleepy brain.
- It's nice to lie in bed and watch the telly, but it can affect your sleep. Try not to do anything too stimulating in bed (apart from sex which can help you to fall asleep).

- Your GP may prescribe a short course of sleeping tablets or other medication (just to help you regain your normal sleep pattern).
- Insomnia can really get people down and many end up dreading going to bed. There are organisations that can help (see the Resource section).
- Those working night shifts can help themselves by aiming to have at least four hours' sleep at the same time every night/morning (e.g. 5–9am). This helps to keep your sleep clock regular. This clock is regulated by light and dark, so take a tip from the vampires and try to get home before sunrise (or put your sunglasses on).

Tip

If you can bear it, try eating a banana, yeast extract and lettuce sandwich for supper. All contain natural substances that help induce sleep.

Point to Ponder

Lie on your bed and take a good look around your bedroom. Does it feel comfortable and inviting? Are there any small changes that would make it feel more so?

Exercise

I feel a bit of a hypocrite writing about the virtues of exercise. It is something that I know I would benefit from, but it has always felt like a very difficult thing to get into. I blame school and the humiliation of always being picked last for team sports! However, exercise does help to speed up the metabolism, which in turn rids the body of excessive levels of stress hormones while increasing the levels of 'feel-good' endorphins. Effective exercise can come for free, e.g. walking up the stairs instead of using the lift or visiting a person in their office instead of phoning them.

A Word of Caution

Before embarking on any new form of exercise it is advisable to discuss it with your GP (especially if you have not taken any exercise for a long time).

Meditation, yoga and visualisation

All of these activities can provide relaxation and a quiet space. While you can teach yourself, it is probably better to find a good teacher (see Resource section).

A really stressed person will usually tell you (and themselves) that they are far too busy to have a hobby. Anyone who really enjoys a hobby will tell you that they are a good activity in which to 'lose yourself'.

Point to Ponder

What hobbies have you done in the past and enjoyed? Might you want to rediscover them? What else interests you?

As the Irish proverb goes – 'A good *laugh* and a long sleep are the best cures in the doctor's book', but what would you think if instead of giving you a prescription for sleeping tablets, your GP gave you two tickets to watch the filming of your favourite comedy show. While this is highly unlikely to happen, research has shown that laughter reduces levels of adrenaline and cortisol (two of the hormones involved in the stress response) and increases endorphin levels. We know that the ability to find humour in a stressful situation has always been a good way of defusing it. Robert Holden, a psychologist and psychotherapist has worked extensively with NHS staff to promote laughter as a stress buster (see Resource section).

Tip

Look in the Resource section for some useful self-help organisations.

Did You Know?

One in 100 adults report that they sleepwalk.

It's a Myth

Older people do not need less sleep, just fewer periods of deep sleep.

Seeking professional help

My routines come out of total unhappiness. My audiences are my group therapy.
Joan Rivers

When stress levels feel huge, you are overly anxious or depressed, and your inner resources and social support are not enough, maybe it's time to seek professional help.

I want to comment on two professional services that I know can be very helpful to people experiencing stress: the general practitioner and the counsellor.

Your GP can be a great ally in helping you to maintain emotional wellbeing, offering support, advice and referral to NHS counselling, psychological and psychiatric services. In addition or instead of, they can offer 'psychoactive medication', usually in the form of antidepressants or anxiolytics. Anything with the word 'psycho' in it can seem daunting and has unfortunate connotations, but all it means is 'the mind'. Although having been around for several decades, these forms of medication are still regarded by many with suspicion. Older readers may remember the use of amphetamines and other drugs that had terrible side effects and were highly addictive. Medicine has come a long way since then. Today, there is a far wider range of medication available and so choice can be more closely tailored to the individual and their needs. Side effects have been reduced and drugs are far more safe and effective than they used to be. While I would never try to persuade someone to take medication if they didn't want to, I have seen some real success stories.

Here are some concerns that people have expressed to me.

- 'I've read some terrible stories in the press about people committing suicide after taking antidepressants.' While these cases are tragic, this kind of reaction to medication is very rare. Ask your GP or pharmacist for further information.
- 'I might get addicted.' GPs are very aware of people's concerns about this and while *some* people can develop a dependence on *some* of the medication, your GP should monitor you closely. Many of the concerns are a throwback to the 1960s and 1970s when people were put on to certain medications to help them cope with a short-term crisis and years later were still on them. Ask your GP or pharmacist to give you information on the possibilities of any dependency that may arise.
- 'I'm frightened that I won't be in control of my faculties.' The Drug Information Sheet will give you details of any potential side effects. Some people find it useful to take the first dose on a day when it doesn't really matter if they feel a little bit drowsy or light-headed and when they don't have to drive or operate machinery. Discuss this with your GP.
- 'What will people think if they know that I'm taking these drugs?' Do people need to know?

If you do decide to accept psychoactive medication from your GP:

- read the drug information sheet that will accompany your medication and discuss any concerns with your GP or pharmacist
- take it as prescribed by your GP. Don't take more (in order to feel better quicker – it won't work and you might harm yourself)
- be aware that, depending on what the drug is, it may take up to three weeks to begin to take effect (although you will feel the benefit of some almost immediately)
- side effects (if any) are usually short-lived and tolerable, but if not, talk to your GP, who may offer you an alternative drug or dose
- don't stop taking the tablets just as you begin to feel better. Again it depends on what you have been prescribed, but most need to be taken for a while after things pick up and withdrawn gradually and under medical supervision. Discuss it with your GP.

Did You Know?

Sixty-six percent of British adults have experienced depression.[9]

Now, let's move on to look at counselling. It can be a daunting thing to embark on counselling so I've put together some information that you may find useful.

Counselling provides an opportunity to talk in confidence to a person who will listen carefully to what you say without judging you. Counsellors are trained to support you through difficult times and help you to make decisions, to solve problems, cope with change, make sense and understand yourself and various situations.

Counsellors do not usually give advice but will provide you with a place where you can discuss your concerns without feeling that you are a burden or that what you say will shock, upset or embarrass.

Counselling can take place individually, in a group, couple or family, face to face, via the telephone, via email or online.

As yet, counselling is an unregulated profession, i.e. there is nothing to stop anyone offering 'counselling'. Some will have no qualification, others a limited amount. An increasing number of counsellors are undergoing a process of accreditation by their professional organisation. Professionally trained counsellors will usually follow a code of ethics or ethical framework.

You can access counselling via:

- your GP
- your occupational health service
- any Employee Assistance Programme (EAP) that your work runs (free to employees)
- voluntary agencies
- some churches and spiritual groups.

Alternatively, you can contact a counsellor who works in private practice near you.

To find contact details of counsellors:

- contact the professional bodies that represent counselling (see Resource section)
- look in the telephone directories
- ask the Citizens Advice Bureau
- consult your local library notice board or database.

Tip

Personal recommendation is a useful way to find a good counsellor.

Counselling is an investment of your time, emotional energy and possibly money. Like any other investment, it is important to choose with care. Most counsellors will provide important information during the first session but if not, it is important to ask about:

- their qualifications, e.g. have they got a Diploma in Counselling or equivalent?
- their experience
- any accreditation that they may have
- any membership of a professional body
- any code of ethics or ethical framework to which they subscribe
- their insurance cover
- fees and cancellation policy
- frequency, length and location of sessions

- number of sessions available
- confidentiality (see below)
- supervision or consultative support (all counsellors should discuss their work with at least one other counsellor)
- the ending process
- referral (who they know that could help if they are unable to).

You don't need to make a decision there and then. You may wish to go away and think through how you felt while talking to this person. Did you feel really listened to? Did they understand (or at least begin to understand) your situation and concerns? Do you think that given time, you would be able to trust them and open up more deeply? If the answer is 'No', discuss your concerns at your next meeting or if you don't think that things could improve, look around for another counsellor.

Signs that the counselling process is not going well.

- The counsellor tells you in great depth about their own problems. NB Some calculated degree of self-disclosure can be part of the therapeutic process.
- They change the fee without discussion with you or without a reasonable amount of notice and discussion with you.
- They cancel appointments without good reason.
- They suggest that you form an additional type of relationship, e.g. become a friend or lover.

Some frequently asked questions (FAQs) about counselling

Q: *Why do people need counsellors? Haven't they got any friends that they can talk to?*
A: Some people don't and this may be part of their underlying concerns. Friends may find it difficult, embarrassing or upsetting to hear intimate details about you; they are too closely involved with you and your life. Even with the best intentions, most friends will, eventually turn the conversation around to their concerns. Sometimes, we don't want to burden our friends or we are worried that they will judge us. They get fed up listening to us. Also, friends have a habit of saying 'If I were you ...'. Will friends always keep your secrets safe?

Q: *Will it be confidential?*
A: Counselling is mainly confidential although there are some exceptions. Although counsellors are required to discuss their work with another counsellor (in supervision) identifying details are not given. Your counsellor should give you further information on confidentiality and supervision during your first session.

Q: *I've heard that there is always a long waiting list for counselling.*
A: That depends on where you go for counselling. For lower-cost or free counselling there may be a waiting list, as there may be to get counselling through the NHS (although not always). Counselling via an EAP or with a counsellor in private practice can usually be arranged quite quickly.

Q: *My GP has given me antidepressants. Can I use counselling at the same time?*
A: In most cases, yes. In some cases of moderate anxiety or depression, it may help to be on the medication for a little while before beginning counselling.

That way, you will be able to use it more effectively. Always tell your counsellor if you are on any medication.

Q: *I sometimes have problems with childcare. If my 3-year-old daughter sits quietly and plays with her jigsaw, can she come to the session with me?*

A: The time in the counselling session is yours to use without distraction. No matter how well behaved your daughter is, she will inevitably take yours and the counsellor's attention away from the process. The counsellor and you may feel inhibited in what is said. Also, think about your daughter, how might she feel if you begin to cry or get angry in the session? Remember that children (even the very young ones) can be very good at picking up bits of information (and sometimes revealing them at a later date).

Q: *I'm very busy. It would be easier (in terms of time) if the counsellor were to see me in my own home? Is this possible?*

A: Some bereavement agencies and other specialist counsellors will counsel in a client's home, but as a rule (and unless there is a special need), counselling usually occurs in a dedicated counselling room.

Q: *I'm on a tight budget. Can I get low-cost or free counselling anywhere?*

A: Yes. Some voluntary counselling agencies offer low-cost or free counselling. Counselling via your GP is also likely to be free (but not always). Counselling via an EAP should be free to employees. Some counsellors in private practice offer a sliding scale.

Q: *English is not my first language. Will a counsellor be able to understand me?*

A: You may decide that in order to convey the exact meaning of what you want to say, you wish to converse in your own language. The professional organisations listed in the Resource section may be able to give you details of counsellors who speak your language.

Tip

More information about counselling can be found in the Resource section.

Point to Ponder

If a colleague told you that they were having counselling, what would be your response?

It's a Myth

There is nothing mysterious about counselling. While it can have hugely positive effects on a person's life, counselling is an ordinary and down-to-earth process.

Did You Know?

Ninety-four percent of people who participated in counselling or psychotherapy would recommend it to others.[9]

References

1 World Health Organization Constitution as adopted by the International Health Conference, New York, 19 June–22 July 1946; signed on 22 July 1946 by the representatives of 61 States (Official Records of the World Health Organization, no. 2, p. 100) and entered into force on 7 April 1948.

2 HSE. *Labour Force Survey: working days lost.* 2004/05 survey of self-reported work-related illness (SWI04/05); 2005.

3 Lazarus RS. *Psychological Stress and the Coping Process.* New York: McGraw-Hill; 1966.

4 Palmer S. Occupational stress. *The Health and Safety Practitioner.* 1989; **7**(8): 16–18.

5 Holmes T and Rahe R The social readjustment rating scale. *Psychosomatic Medicine.* 1967; **11**: 213–18.

6 Maslach C, Jackson SE. The measurement of experienced burnout. *J Occup Behav.* 1981; **2**: 99–113.

7 Goldberg N. *Wild Mind: living the writer's life.* New York: Bantam; 1990.

8 Porter EH. *Pollyanna.* Wordsworth Childrens Classics. Hertfordshire: Wordsworth Editions; 1994.

9 Mintel/YouGov Report, April 2006.

Chapter 11

Understanding yourself

The importance of self-understanding

I have often wished I had time to cultivate modesty... But I am too busy thinking about myself.

Edith Sitwell

What is it like to be you? What do you know about your motives, fears, hopes, prejudices, drives, influences, attitudes, thoughts, patterns, traits, values, feelings, behaviour and decisions? And, very important in the healthcare professions, what do you know about how you relate to people? Self-understanding (or self-awareness) is not just an intellectual exercise. It is about noticing your own existence, what is happening inside of you, between other people and you, and you 'in the world'.

Looking at our own identity requires courage, honesty and compassion. Healthcare is a demanding profession and one in which we must have a strong sense of who we are if people are to see us as confident, competent and reliable. Without a good understanding of who we are, we run the risk of focusing all our attention on others while walking around in what seems like another person's body and mind.

Many people have genuine concerns about looking more closely at themselves, describing it as 'navel gazing', 'self-indulgent' and 'attention seeking'. For one thing, it is your navel to gaze at if you so choose. Second, what is wrong (particularly in your profession) with giving yourself some attention. As the proverb goes: *When everyone takes care of himself, care is taken of all.*

A common argument against seeking to increase your self-understanding comes from the 'best left well alone' brigade. At some time in their lives, most people have learnt to avoid seeing parts of themselves. Maybe these parts were unacceptable to those whose approval we sought. From a very young age most of us began to mould ourselves into what was expected. Along the way, bits of us got shut away in boxes and put high on a shelf. The problem is that every so often (and without warning or apparent cause), one of these boxes falls from the shelf, comes open and spills its contents all over our lives and relationships. If you can guarantee that none of your boxes will ever fall off the shelf then there is no need to look any deeper into yourself.

So how do you work out how much you already know about yourself? You could sit down and to some degree work it out by asking yourself questions such as 'What do I like about myself?', 'How do I respond when under pressure?' or 'How do I react to authority figures'. You *could* do it that way but given that the list of questions is probably endless and perhaps more importantly, it is a lonely task, you could try another way. The Johari Window (Figure 11.1) is a

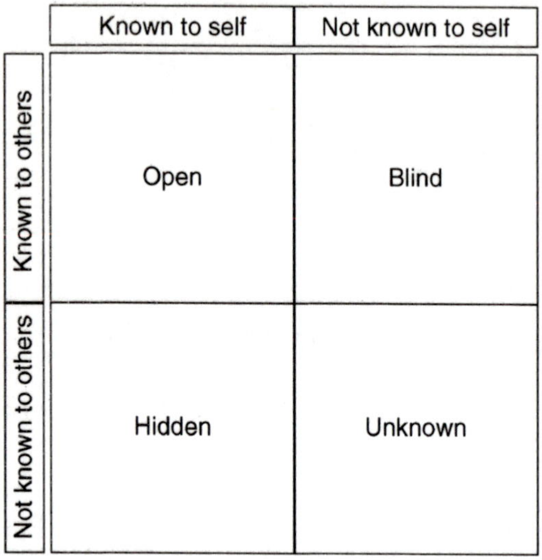

	Known to self	Not known to self
Known to others	Open	Blind
Not known to others	Hidden	Unknown

Figure 11.1 The Johari Window.

simple and useful way of helping people to: (a) assess how much they already know about themselves; and (b) learn some more.[1]

I'm starting from the assumption that the human mind is made up of conscious and unconscious parts, each containing information about us. The Johari Window divides this information into four different types, as represented by the panes of a window.

- The *open* area contains information known to me and known to other people, e.g. friends, colleagues, relatives. For example, I know that I like chocolate (and a lot of people know that about me too).
- The *blind* area contains information that others can see about me but I can't, e.g. I don't realise it, but other people have noticed that I've got chocolate stains down my white jumper.
- The *hidden* area contains information that I know about myself but choose not to reveal to others, e.g. perhaps I eat two family-sized bars of chocolate each day (and more at weekends).
- The *unknown* area contains information that neither I nor others know, e.g. my mother used to give me chocolate buttons whenever I was upset. So while I don't realise it, I must be feeling upset most of the time to comfort myself with so much chocolate.

The golden rule about the Johari Window is that while its overall size never changes, the size of the window panes can. If one expands, another has to shrink to accommodate the change.

The *open* area can never shrink, i.e. a friend can never 'unlearn' something about me. It grows when I disclose further information about myself. As a consequence, the hidden area shrinks. The *blind* area can never grow. It shrinks when I receive feedback about myself from others. The *hidden* area becomes smaller when I make self-disclosures and as a result the open area increases in size. The *unknown* area can never become bigger. It lessens in size when I gain information and insights from my unconscious.

The Johari Window should be handled with care. Self-disclosure can be a tricky business. If you want to tell your secrets to someone, choose that person very carefully. The aim of the disclosure is to gain some insight into your own mind, not to provide gossip for others. Some secrets are best kept that way.

Remember that the blind area contains information that you don't yet know. When asking for feedback from others, ask someone you can trust to be truthful and sensitive (rather than someone who will see it as a chance to have a go at you). Hold in mind that feedback is just another person's view (and not carved in stone); you can choose to accept or reject it. If you feel unsure, ask for more information, clarification or examples. You can also ask someone else for a second opinion.

A Word of Caution

Any person's 'unknown area' *could* include very sensitive material arising from early events or traumatic times that has been filed away to protect the conscious mind. If you know or suspect that this may be case for you, it is best to work on your unknown area within a therapeutic setting, e.g. with a counsellor or psychotherapist.

Experiment

Draw three boxes and label them Open, Blind and Hidden. Go through the following list and choose words that describe you. Now, ask someone whose opinion you value to go down the same list, choosing words that *they* think apply to you. Afterwards, write words that you have *both* chosen in the Open box, words that only *you* have chosen in the Hidden box and words that only your *friend* has chosen in the Blind box.

Loving	Calm	Confident	Proud	Risk taking
Caring	Angry	Sad	Intelligent	Organised
Responsible	Happy	Introvert	Anxious	Patient
Generous	Neat	Funny	Chaotic	Excitable
Serious	Methodical	Friendly	Dependable	Extrovert

Transactional Analysis is another way of looking at yourself and how you relate to other people. Developed by Eric Berne, a 20th-century psychiatrist, this is a very accessible model and one that has helped a lot of people to understand more about themselves and their relationships. In essence, we all have ego states (patterns of thinking, feeling and behaving). There are three, but only one of these ego states will be in charge of who we are at any one moment.[2]

- Adult ego state – the part of us that can organise, make objective judgements, apply intelligence and logic.
- Parent ego state – feelings, thoughts, behaviours and attitudes of a parental figure or role.
- Child ego state – feelings, thoughts, behaviours and attitudes of a child ('childlike' rather than 'childish').

The parent ego state can be further divided into two parts: the critical or controlling parent (which is rule driven) and the nurturing parent (who takes care of). The child ego state can also be divided into two parts: the adapted child (overly compliant 'good boy' or rebellious 'bad boy') and the free or natural child (spontaneous, fun-loving, creative).

Each part can manifest itself at any time and in any situation (both appropriately and inappropriately). While it is acceptable and appropriate for me to boo the villain at a pantomime, it would be inappropriate for me to boo a colleague with whom I disagreed during a business meeting. Similarly, it may be appropriate for me to speak in nurturing tones when my partner is unwell but not to 'mummy' him by making sure that he cleans his teeth properly each day. At work it is generally considered appropriate to be in our adult ego state (unless our work role dictates otherwise, e.g. playing with children).

We can flip very quickly between one ego state and another; sometimes on purpose and at other times without realising it. Occasionally, the ego of one person will trigger a change in that of another person. For example, I may be feeling very 'critical parent' towards my son who has left his toys all over the floor (again), but when he throws his arms around me and tell me that he loves me, my ego state changes to one of 'nurturing parent'.

The key to this is becoming aware of your own ego states (and observing those of others). That way, we know where we are 'coming from' and 'going to'.

Tip

Maturity is not about getting rid of the child part from us, but allowing each ego state to become evident when appropriate.

Points to Ponder

- Do you recognise any of these ego states in (a) yourself and (b) others?
- Do you feel more at home in one ego state than another?
- What ego state do you inhabit at work?
- In which different ego states do you see patients and relatives (and under what situations)?
- What is your attitude to self-exploration?
- Do you know anyone with whom you can discuss yourself in an honest and open way?

Who Said This?

Which member of The Goons was the first man to appear on the cover of *Playboy* and said: 'There is no me. I do not exist. There used to be a me but I had it surgically removed':

(a) Spike Milligan?
(b) Harry Secombe?
(c) Peter Sellers?

Did You Know?

Functional magnetic resonance imaging suggests that the part of the brain responsible for self-awareness is called the superfrontal gyrus.[3] This brain structure is located behind the forehead (the same part of the head that people sometimes slap when something has just occurred to them).

There are many different ways to increase your self-understanding and the next section offers you information about some of these ways.

Learning more about yourself

There came a time when the risk to remain tight in the bud was more painful than the risk it took to blossom.

Anaïs Nin

My only regret in life is that I am not someone else.

Woody Allen

There are many ways that you can increase your self-understanding. The internet, libraries, bookshops and bookshelves across the world are packed with ways that claim to advance personal understanding. While many are sensible, tried-and-tested methods that have worked for lots people over the years, others are more, shall I say... on the edge.

Here are a selection of ways that I have used to help people learn more about themselves (including myself):

- noticing yourself more
- reading and the arts
- keeping a reflective journal
- free-drawing
- making a life line
- using your imagination
- counselling.

Noticing yourself more

Noticing yourself is the key to self-understanding and a skill that develops over time and with practice. There are many aspects of yourself that you can notice. Here are two to begin with.

1 How you do use language? Notice how often you use 'should', 'ought' and 'must'. These are order or directive type words that can give you clues about the 'early messages' that you received and still give yourself, e.g. 'I must not waste time'. How many times do you say 'I have to...' (an inner command) rather than 'I want to...' (which has more personal power). Similarly, 'I can't' versus 'I won't'. Information gained from noticing your use of language will enable you to make choices.

2 How much do you tune in to your body? While you may be aware of which bits hurt and ache, what do you know about the rest of it? Which bits tingle, feel tense, hot or ignored? Scanning your body from toes to head can give you information about how you really are and what your body might need.

Reading and the arts

Your local bookshop is likely to have a wide selection of 'self-help' books, many claiming to have the answer to life's problems, questions and concerns. While some self-help books are useful, many are not; but how do you tell? One way is to go by personal recommendation from someone whose opinion you value. Another way is to notice the image the book is attempting to portray: does it promote a 'get-well-quick' approach, 'overnight enlightenment', have glossy images and lots of smiley people? You are only likely to benefit from a book if it is written in a style and uses language that you can understand (rather than jargon or impressive-sounding psychobabble). It may seem obvious, but if a book is to have any chance of helping you, it has to be read. Many people tell me about the shelves and shelves of self-help books in their home, all in perfect condition and none of them read.

Various authors, poets, film makers, musicians and artists have produced works that have helped people to understand themselves, other people and life a little bit more, e.g. Tolstoy, George Eliot, Alice Walker, DH Lawrence, Doris Lessing, Harper Lee, Michelangelo, Vaughan Williams, Reginald Rose, Hitchcock, Viktor Frankl, CS Lewis, TS Eliot.

Keeping a reflective journal

Some people find that writing material about themselves can benefit self-understanding. Reflective journals are usually written without regard to grammar, spelling or neatness. The more we try to 'do it right' the more likely we are to censor what we write. Just noticing how you use the journal can be revealing in itself. Although it is useful to write an entry each day, it should not become a chore. Although you may wish to record the day's events (and this is a good place to start), the emphasis is more on your inner experience, your thoughts, feelings, imaginings, dreams, daydreams and insights. From time to time, it is useful to review your journal, noting any themes and realisations. While reflective journals are usually private, you may wish to share some of the contents with a trusted friend.

Free-drawing

Drawing is a good way of accessing, clarifying and expressing our thoughts and feelings. Like journal writing, it is not about getting it right, nor does it involve being artistic. Use coloured pencils or, even better, crayons, and give yourself enough room to draw. It may help to sit on the floor rather than at a table. This technique is called 'free drawing' because the emphasis is on allowing ideas to filter through rather than thinking what colour or shape something 'should be'.

When you have finished your drawing, stand back from it. Don't try to interpret it but just notice things about it.

Case Study

During Oliver's appraisal, his manager had commented on his lack of assertiveness when dealing with elderly male patients. He tended to let them walk all over him. At home, Oliver decided to draw himself and some of the male patients that he knew. When he looked at his drawing he noticed that all of the patients appeared to be bigger then him (which was odd because Oliver was over 6 feet tall). He also noticed that he had arranged the patients in a circle around him. As he looked deeper into his drawing, he was reminded of times when as a child, his four older brothers would stand around him and make bullying and taunting comments. Oliver could never escape from them and the only way that he could end the experience was to keep quiet until they became bored and went away. By free drawing, Oliver was able to make links between his experience as a child and how he now related to older men.

Like journal writing, free drawing is usually a solitary activity, but some people do find it useful to show their drawing to a trusted friend who can add comments and observations. Doing 'free drawing' with another person can also help if you wish to understand your relationship more deeply.

Making a life line

A life line is a way to represent your life and the events that have helped shape you. You will need a roll of paper (perhaps old wallpaper) or simply some sheets of plain paper stuck together. Draw on the plain side, a long, straight line and mark out your life in terms of years. It seems logical to start at your birth and end at the age that you are now, but some people start the line before they were born or even before they were conceived. They see the events that preceded their arrival as significant to the path of their life. Like the start of the life line and depending on your spiritual outlook, you may wish to continue the line after the point that you speculate could be the end of your physical existence.

Then, mark along the line major events that have occurred in your life and that feel significant to you, e.g. broke arm, went to school, sister born, failed 11+, began puberty, took exams, left school, started first job, got sacked, got married, had first baby, mother died, got divorced…, etc. Write in events that are planned for or could occur in the future. Take a step back and look at your life line as a whole. What do you see? What strikes you? Do any patterns or themes emerge? Have you missed out anything important? What might that mean to you? How have you changed as time has passed? What have you achieved? What major decisions were made or not made? What paths did you choose? What might have been? Would you have liked your life to have been any different? How would you like your life to be in the future? Are there still opportunities? Again, this is an activity that you can do alone or with another trusted friend.

At the end of your life line, you may wish to imagine a scene surrounding your funeral. Who would be there and what tributes might they pay to you? What would be written on your gravestone?

Using your imagination

Freud called dreams, 'the royal road to the unconscious'. Some people say that they never dream, others do but quickly forget the dream and a few remember dreams for years. Sometimes we have a dream that stays with us throughout the day and feels significant in some way. These are not necessarily (and often not) nightmares, but what Freud called 'big dreams'. Sometimes, people say that the dream seemed to be speaking to them (even though the 'message' was not clear). The meaning of the dream may arrive on waking, hours, days or years later, or never. To be able to use the message from a dream does not require a conscious link between the message and the dream.

There are various ways that you can use your dreams to understand yourself more.

- You can record dreams in a 'dream diary' or reflective journal; the feelings, emotions, colours, characters, oddities or whatever occurs to you. Do any themes emerge? Does anything strike you as unusual or strange, e.g. are there any obvious omissions or contradictions? Could the dream hold a message?
- Another way is to describe your dream as if it were happening now. Use the present tense, e.g. 'I am walking down the tree-lined avenue. I see a brown dog near the road'. Describe how you are feeling in the dream, e.g. 'I am feeling worried as I see the dog running into the road'. How do you feel as you describe the scene? What might it be telling you about yourself?
- Sometimes the unconscious looks at things in a back-to-front way, i.e. it gives you a dream that features the opposite of what it might want your conscious mind to do. For example, a woman who dreams that she stabbed her best friend's husband may, in the 'back of her mind', harbour fantasies of an illicit affair.

Don't try to over-analyse your dreams. If you don't get the message first time, your ingenious unconscious will relay it to you another night, in a different way.

I don't find 'dream dictionaries' useful, e.g. to dream that you have broken your leg means that you will inherit some money. Only you can make definitive interpretations of your dream symbols.

Apart from its relaxing effects, *meditation* can be another way towards greater self-understanding. Although sometimes shrouded in mystique, meditation really is quite ordinary. During a meditative state, the metabolism and levels of chemicals associated with stress, decrease. While a meditator is fully awake and able to respond to any emergency or call from 'the outside', there is a sense of slowing down and hibernation. Brain waves change from the faster beta to the slower alpha brain waves. Brain activity moves its emphasis from the left side of the brain (associated with the logical, rational, analytical thinking) to the right side (associated with intuition, feelings, looking at the bigger picture).

The ability to distance yourself from the busyness and demands of everyday living can be extremely restorative and provides a space for you to tune into yourself. Although it can take time to learn how to meditate effectively, it requires no special clothes or equipment and can be done in a group or alone. You can teach yourself how to meditate (using books, tapes or DVDs) or you can find a teacher who will help you.

Word of Caution

Choose a meditation teacher with care. See the Resource section for further information.

'Mandy, stop staring out of the window and pay attention, girl...!', 'If Clive would stop daydreaming, he could go far...' – typical phrases from schooldays. From a very early age we are actively encouraged to 'stay on task' and 'pay attention'. While I am not denying that to succeed and be safe in the world we must be in contact with what is going on around us, activities like *daydreaming* are not encouraged. Daydreaming is turning attention away from a focus, a physical or mental task. By doing this, we can create an uncluttered space that has potential and can be likened to a 'holiday for the mind and body', a reverie. During a daydream, our sense of time can change, e.g. what seems like 30 minutes may only be 30 seconds. During daydreaming, the brain waves change from the faster beta to slower alpha waves and activity switches from left to right brain. Of course, some people take daydreaming to an extreme, often as a way to escape the demands and responsibilities of relationships and life. Again, it is a matter of balance.

Counselling

The previous section covered counselling in some detail. Exploring yourself with someone who is otherwise not involved in your life can be a great way of helping you to understand yourself more. You don't need to have 'a problem' to be able to approach a counselling service or to use it effectively.

Who Said This?

Which famous American actress starred in *Gentleman Prefer Blondes* and said: 'I always felt I was a nobody, and the only way for me to be somebody was to be – well, somebody else. Which is probably why I wanted to act':

(a) Lauren Bacall?
(b) Marilyn Monroe?
(c) Betty Grable?

Tips

Remember, increasing your self-understanding need not involve money. Beware sources of help that make big claims and guarantee success. Personal recommendation from a friend or trusted colleague can be invaluable.

References

1 Luft J, Ingham H. The Johari window, a graphic model of interpersonal awareness. *Proceedings of the Western Training Laboratory in Group Development*. Los Angeles: UCLA; 1955.
2 Berne E. *Games People Play*. New York: Grove Press; 1964.
3 Golderg, I, Harel M, Malach R. When the brain loses its self: prefrontal inactivation during sensorimotor processing. *Neuron*. 2006; **50**(2): 329–39.

Final thoughts

I hope that you have enjoyed reading this book. It has been a real pleasure and privilege to write.

I have often thought of it as a baby: imagined, created, shaped, loved and very occasionally, loathed. Now, it is time for the baby to leave home. While I will have more free time and space for other important things and people, I am very aware of the void that its departure is likely to leave in my life (at least for a while). Perhaps this mirrors the conflicting thoughts and ambivalent feelings that many healthcare workers have about *their* work.

While writing, I have very much focused on *you* as a person, as well as an employee. Working with people is not easy. If we are to do a good enough job each day *and* remain resilient, we must bring to it our humanity and understanding.

My hope is that this book goes some way towards helping and supporting you in your work and elsewhere.

Resources

Chapter 1

Kratz DM. *Effective Listening Skills: business skills express*. Chicago, IL: Irwin Professional; 1995.

Sanders P, editor. *First Steps in Counselling*. 2nd ed. Ross-on-Wye: PCCS Books; 1996.

Summerfield J, van Oudtshoorn L. *Counselling in the Workplace*. London: Institute of Personnel and Development; 1995.

Theobald T, Cooper C. *Shut Up and Listen!: the truth about how to communicate at work*. London: Kogan Page; 2004.

Chapter 2

Faulkner A. *When the News is Bad: a guide for health professionals*. Cheltenham: Stanley Thorne; 1998.

The following organisations offer useful information on mental health conditions:

The Royal College of Psychiatrists
Tel: 020 7245 1231
Email: rcpsych@rcpsych.ac.uk
Website: www.rcpsych.ac.uk

MIND
Tel: 0845 766 0163
Website: www.mind.org.uk

SANE
Tel: 020 7375 1002
Email: London@sane.org.uk
Website: www.sane.org.uk

SANELINE is a helpline offering practical information, crisis care and emotional support to anyone affected by mental health issues. Tel: 0845 767 8000 (1–11pm).

Chapter 3

Dryden W. *Assertiveness Step by Step*. London: Sheldon Press; 2004.
Lilley R. *Dealing with Difficult People*. London: Kogan Page; 2002.

ACAS
Tel: 08457 474747.
Website: www.acas.org.uk
Offers information and training regarding workplace issues and difficulties.

Further information on the Healthcare Commission is available on www.healthcarecommission.org.uk.

Chapter 4

Hooker J. *Working Across Cultures*. Stanford, CA: Stanford University Press; 2003.
Lustig M, Koester J. *Intercultural Competence: interpersonal communication across cultures*.
    Boston, MA: Allyn & Bacon; 2005.

Royal National Institute for the Deaf
Tel: 0808 808 0123
Textphone: 0808 808 900
Email: informationline@rnid.org.uk
Website: www.rnid.org.uk

Royal National Institute for the Blind
Tel: 020 7388 1266
Helpline: 0845 766 9999 (Mon–Fri, 9am–5pm)
Email: helpline@rnib.org.uk
Website: www.rnib.org.uk

Commission for Racial Equality
Website: www.cre.gov.uk

Disability Rights Commission
Tel: 08457 622 633
Textphone: 08457 622 644
Website: www.drc-gb.org

For a glossary of medical terms related to communication disorders, see www.wikipedia.org.

Geert Hofstede
www.geerthofstede.nl

Chapter 5

Forsyth P. *Telephone Skills* (Management Shapers). London: Chartered Institute of Personnel
    and Development; 2000.
Kratz DM. *Effective Listening Skills: business skills express*. Chicago, IL: Irwin Professional;
    1995.
Sanders P., editor. *An Incomplete Guide to Using Counselling Skills on the Telephone* (revised
    2e). Manchester: PCCS; 1996.
Smith H. *Letter Writing, E-mail and Texting* (Essentials). Berkshire: Foulsham; 2003.

Chapter 6

Brown CL. *Essential Delegation Skills*. The Smart Management Guide Series. Hampshire:
    Gower Publishing; 1997.
Perry A. *Isn't It About Time?: how to overcome procrastination and get on with your life*. London:
    Worth Publishing; 2002.

Chapter 7

Buzan T. *The Ultimate Book of Mind Maps*. London; Harper Thorsons; 2006.
de Bono E. *Lateral Thinking: a textbook of creativity*. London: Penguin Books; 1990.
Jones M. *The Thinker's Toolkit: 14 powerful techniques for problem solving*. Emeryville, CA:
    Three Rivers Press; 1998.
Storey R. *The Influencing Pocketbook*. Hampshire: Management Pocketbooks; 2000.

Chapter 8

Covey SR. *The 7 Habits of Highly Effective People*. London; Simon and Schuster UK; 1989.
Pincus M, Miller R. *Running a Meeting that Works*. New York: Barron's Educational Series; 2004.

Chapter 9

Poertner S, Miller KM. *The Art of Giving and Receiving Feedback* (Communication Skills. S). Boulder, CA: American Media Inc.; 1996.
Thorn J. *How to Negotiate Better Deals*. London: Mercury Books; 1991.

Mediation UK is a national voluntary organisation dedicated to developing constructive means of resolving conflicts in communities. Website: www.mediationuk.org.uk.

Chapter 10

Adler A. *What Life Could Mean To You*. Oxford: OneWorld; 1998.
Bristow W. *The Art of the Daydream*. London: MQ Publications; 2004.
Bryant-Jefferies R. *A little Book of Therapy*. Brighton: Pen Press; 2006.
Bunting M. *Willing Slaves – how to overcome culture in ruling our lives*. London: Harper Collins; 2004.
de Bono E. *Lateral Thinking: a textbook of creativity*. London: Penguin Books; 1990.
de Bono E. *De Bono's Thinking Course*. London: BBC Active; 2004.
Harris C. *Minimise Stress, Maximise Success: how to rise above it all and realise your goals*. London: Duncan Baird; 2003.
Macmahon G. *How to Make Life Happen: when you're too busy to live*. London: Sheldon Press; 2006.
Pines A., Aronson E., editors. *Career Burnout: causes and cures*. 2nd ed. New York: Free Press; 1988.
TUC. *Keeping Well at Work – a TUC guide*. 2nd ed. London: Kogan Page; 2001.

WorkLifeBalanceCentre
Tel: 01530 273 056
Website: www.worklifebalancecentre.org

NHS Direct
Tel: 0845 4647
Website: www.nhsdirect.co.uk

Information about counselling and psychotherapy plus lists of practitioners:

British Association for Counselling and Psychotherapy (BACP)
Tel: 0870 443 5252
Email: bacp@bacp.co.uk
Website: www.bacp.co.uk

UK Council for Psychotherapy (UKCP)
Tel: 020 7014 9955
Email: info@psychotherapy.org.uk
Website: www.ukcp.org.uk

COSCA (Counselling and Psychotherapy in Scotland) accredited
Tel: 01786 475 140
Website: www.cosca.org.uk

Irish Association for Counselling and Psychotherapy
Tel: 00 35 31 230 0061
Email: iacp@irish-counselling.ie
Website: www.irish-counselling.ie

NAFSIYAT Intercultural Therapy Centre
Tel: 020 7686 8666

Pink Therapy (therapy for sexual minority clients)
Tel: 020 7291 4480
Email: info@pinktherapy.com
Website: www.pinktherapy.com

Managing stress:

International Stress Management Association
Tel: 07000 780 430
Website: www.isma.org.uk

Centre for Stress Management
Tel: 020 8228 1185
Website: www.managingstress.com

Carole Spiers Group
Tel: 020 89541593
Email: info@carolespiersgroup.co.uk
Website: www.carolespiersgroup.co.uk

Alcohol:

DrinkAware
Website: www.drinkaware.co.uk

Drugs:

Talk to Frank
Tel: 0800 776600
Website: www.talktofrank.com

Dependence on over-the-counter medication:

Over-Count
9 Croft Road
Bankend Village
Dumfries DG1 4RW
Tel: 01387 770 404

Food and emotional wellbeing:

British Nutrition Foundation
Tel: 020 7404 6504
Email: postbox@nutrition.org.uk
Website: www.nutrition.org.uk

Sleeping well:

The Better Sleep Council
Website: www.bettersleep.org

Laughter and emotional wellbeing:

The Happiness Project
Tel: 0845 430 9236
Email: info@hapiness.co.uk
Website: www.happinessproject.co.uk

Yoga:

The British Wheel of Yoga
Tel: 01529 306 851
Email: office@bwy.org.uk
Website: www.bwy.org.uk

Meditation:

London Buddhist Centre
Tel: 020 8981 1225
Email: info@lbc.org.uk
Website: www.lbc.org.uk

Transcendental Meditation
Tel: 020 7402 3451
Email: mail@tm-london.org.uk
Website: www.tm-london.org.uk

TUC

Campaign for a fair deal at work and for social justice at home and abroad.
Tel: 020 7636 4030
Website: www.tuc.org.uk

The Health and Safety Executive
Tel: 0845 345 0055
Website: www.hse.gov.uk

Chapter 11

Berne E. *Games People Play: the psychotherapy of human relationships*. London: Penguin; 1964.
de Bono E. *How to Have a Beautiful Mind*. London: Vermilion; 2004.
Harris A., Harris T., editors. *Staying OK*. 2nd ed. Ed. London: Pan Books; 1985.
Rowan J. *Discover Your Subpersonalities: our inner world and the people in it*. London: Routledge; 1993.

Answers to 'Who Said This?'

Chapter 1: (a).
Chapter 2: (c).
Chapter 5: (b).
Chapter 6: (a).
Chapter 7: (a).
Chapter 8: (b).
Chapter 9: (c); (a).
Chapter 10: (b).
Chapter 11: (c); (b).

Index